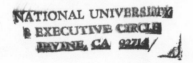

JUMP for JOY

The Rebounding Exercise Book

James R. White, Ph.D.
with Lan Barnes

ARCO PUBLISHING, INC.
NEW YORK

For Raymond E. White and
Zelma LaVon Emerson

Lan Barnes, editor
Margaret Bartlett White, manuscript preparation
Raoul Sudre and Margaret Bartlett White, photographs

Published by Arco Publishing, Inc.
215 Park Avenue South, New York, N.Y. 10003

Library of Congress Cataloging in Publication Data

White, James R., 1932–
  Jump for joy.

  1. Trampolining. 2. Aerobic exercises. 3. Physical
fitness. I. Barnes, Lan. II. Title.
GV555.W48 1983   796.4'7   83-12211
ISBN 0-668-05836-6 (Cloth Edition)
ISBN 0-668-05842-0 (Paper Edition)

Printed in the United States of America

10 9 8 7 6 5 4 3 2 1

Contents

Foreword

A positive attitude toward life must include a positive attitude toward one's health. An astonishing increase in consciousness is evident in the millions of people who exercise regularly. This change in behavior is a true revolution, a turning around of individuals, a manifestation of an inner change that has the effect of altering life-styles.

In Western Europe, this massive change in behavior was seen in the Middle Ages, during the Crusades, when the entire culture was absorbed in the process of "Freeing the Holy Land." The West emerged from the Crusades a changed culture. The passions of the crusading years are part of the heritage of present-day Western ideology.

The intense preoccupation with personal health is another form of crusade. What we are attempting to free is held hostage by the following enemies: sloth, obesity, constriction, and the complex of messages that try to convince us that we are indeed doomed to a perpetual downhill slide into disability, chronic illness and depression. We must use many weapons to liberate ourselves from these oppressive forces. *Jump for Joy* is one such weapon that will go a long way toward assisting us in winning our inner crusade.

The principles of exercise in this book are sound and based upon careful research and observation. Runners, swimmers, hikers, body builders, walkers, bicyclers, tennis players—anyone who has found his or her own personal way to personal freedom—can benefit from this book. And it is an excellent book for any beginner who may be too shy to enter the public arena of exercise.

I recommend it heartily, and wish you many jumps for joy.

THADDEUS KOSTRUBALA, MD

Del Mar, California

Preface

As a health researcher, I'm a little skeptical about a lot of things. The first time I saw "miniature rebounding equipment" I was very skeptical. And as a member of the California Health Fraud Association, I immediately thought, "Oh no, not another gimmick to fool the public."

Curiosity got the best of me, however, and I decided to bring one of those strange "springing devices" into the physical education research laboratory at the University of California, San Diego, and find the truth about the manufacturers' extravagant claim that jumping on rebounding equipment is "the best exercise in the universe."

After three and a half years of extensive research, we found that jumping on rebounding equipment is the best form of exercise for some but not for others.* For most people, it's fine. We found that 93 percent of 2300 men, women and children who jumped in our laboratory experienced a great deal of joy. In fact, there was a smile on everyone's face. From these studies we concluded that jumping on rebounding equipment is a form of exercise that can be used by both novice and expert athletes, weight losers, those with various injuries, jogging dropouts, executives pressed for time, those living in extreme climates and especially those who hate exercise.

Rebounding centers are springing up around the country, but as you might expect, most jumping occurs at home. People are successful at rebounding because it is one exercise that is not painful, inconvenient or boring. We can make these statements based on the results of a two-year study conducted on executives who had completed the Sun Valley Health Institute Fitness Program. Here, the participants chose between outdoor running, indoor stationary bicycling or jumping on rebounding equipment as their main form of exercise.

Jumping was the best form of exercise in terms of how many executives were still exercising after 12 months. Forty-eight percent

*See Medical Applications, pages 189–192.

of the joggers were still running, 17 percent of the cyclists were pedaling, and 76 percent of the jumpers were still at it.

Why did so many remain faithful? The reasons were convenience, availability, weatherproofness, absence of leg trauma, and—probably the most important reason—that it was just plain fun. Some of the executives were marathon racers, some hadn't jogged a step in 30 to 40 years, and some just needed something to do on a rainy afternoon. But all agreed that they could now find time for a little exercise in their lives.

All human beings are similar in some ways, and jumping is a natural expression of joy for everyone. Little children waiting to get on a merry-go-round jump up and down with excitement. At a professional football game, we're used to seeing the 260-pound, macho all-stars bound uninhibitedly into the air following the scoring of the winning touchdown. Jumping offers an important new option in fitness and fun. It is a growing activity and an important part of America's recent fitness renaissance.

During the last decade, we tested and prescribed exercise and nutrition programs for over 8000 people. We tried many types of exercise and used nearly every method to motivate people to begin and continue exercise. For you to succeed, the bottom line is that you must embark on a fitness program that is individualized, convenient and enjoyable.

You probably realize that exercise and fitness are worth experiencing. I want to show you how you can bounce your way to fitness, and I want to give you new ways to measure, achieve and maintain just about any level of fitness you desire. This book covers a variety of topics, but it emphasizes jumping as either the main activity or as a supplement to your present exercise.

Many physicians have expressed an interest in finding out if jumping on rebounding equipment is safe for their patients. We have directed thousands of doctor-referred patients through our program and found that jumping can be safely used for injury prevention and disease rehabilitation, and, combined with proper nutrition, it has proved to be an effective and long-lasting means of weight control. A special section on medical use has been included as an appendix (page 189).

Finally, for you skiers, we've included a program guaranteed to improve your downhill turns. Bouncing on a mini-rebounder—to music—may sound like another "con job," but in the laboratory we found that it works. We think you'll find that jumping will have a permanent, appropriate and joyful place in your future.

Happy jumping!

1

Jumping for Joy—What and Why

A LITTLE HISTORY

In our laboratory at the University of California, San Diego (UCSD), we have undoubtedly heard every excuse for *not* exercising known to man. It's too cold outside, too dark, too dangerous (snarling beasts, autos, smog), too boring, too embarrassing or too hot and humid. We call these the "Terrible Too's."

Well, we've come up with an answer for exercising that is fun, safe and comfortable. It's called "jumping for joy." It's an excellent method of weight control because you can burn off between 5 and 12 calories* per minute, and if you follow a 30- to 40-minute-per-day program, you can easily lose up to 30 pounds of fat per year.

Jumping on rebounding equipment is exercising by jumping, turning, twisting, dancing, doing calisthenics, rope skipping, jogging and practicing downhill skiing. It's best done to music. The rebounding equipment is a simple nylon-floored distant relative to the trampoline, differing in that it is only 3 to 4 feet in size and is raised about 6 to 7 inches from the floor. It is *not* used for flips or other acrobatics.

The bounce adds new dimensions to exercise by making it fun instead of boring, light instead of traumatic, and at the same time produces a thin body and a strong and healthy heart.

---

*When I use the term "calorie" in this book, I always mean the dietitian's (and dieter's) calorie, equal to 1000 of the physicist's calories. But don't be confused; if you have a diet book, calorie means the same thing here as it does there.

Seven years ago we began using rebounding equipment for programs of rehabilitation for students, faculty and staff at UCSD. Some participants had suffered heart attacks or had heart disease; others had injured backs, knees and ankles; and many were simply overweight.

Jumping for rehabilitation proved successful because the bed of the rebounding equipment is very yielding against the striking foot, and virtually nontraumatic as compared to walking or jogging on hard surfaces. The patients exercised for extended periods of time without becoming fatigued. In fact, the rehabilitation was so enjoyable that many chose jumping as their favorite recreational exercise. Many of our patients purchased their own jumper for home use. The activity became so popular on campus that we had to arrange special noon-time classes for secretaries and other faculty and staff. Their fitness improved and their obesity declined.

These clinical observations were substantiated in a study reported at the 1980 American College of Sports Medicine convention in Las Vegas. The study, conducted in this author's laboratory, showed improvement in fitness and reduction in body fat in 70 women after ten weeks of daily exercise on rebounders, improvement that was equivalent to that found following stationary bicycling or treadmill-running programs.

The exercise is "pleasantly fatiguing without joint trauma." It demands a bit of huffing and puffing and has been described as "great fun, but a little work." The amount and intensity of jumping will vary according to your age. Later I will show you how to determine and follow your exercise program at an exact exercise heart rate (Chapter 8).

WHY JUMP FOR JOY?

Have you heard a gentle thud, thud, thud at 6:30 A.M.? It could be the rhythm of a jogger's gait or, if the thuds are heard with music, they could be the ambulations of someone jumping to keep his or her body totally fit, to lose weight, to improve his or her figure, to reduce anxiety, and to increase that overall feeling of well-being.

These are good reasons for exercising—but there are more. Exercise will reduce the chance of, and may even prevent, coronary heart disease. When you jump regularly for a sufficient length of time, every cell in your body changes and improves. A major change is that the oxygen in the air you breathe is more efficiently transported into the blood stream and is more effectively used by the muscles. In addition, the heart becomes stronger and is better able to supply greater amounts of blood to the lungs and working muscles.

The basic physiological changes go by a variety of names: "cardiovascular enhancement," "increased aerobic capacity," "the training effect," "improved stamina," "endurance," or "improved wind." I don't care what you call it, I know that jumping will provide you with greater physical fitness and health—that's the bottom line.

Jumping is considered *aerobic* exercise because it uses large muscles in a rhythmic manner and is performed over a period of 10 to 40 minutes. An opposite form of exercise is *anaerobic* exercise, which is characterized by short, forceful and near-maximal movements that may place additional stress on the heart and afford little or no benefits to the heart.

Aerobic-rhythmical exercise includes jogging, running, bicycling, swimming, skating, cross-country skiing and jumping. Aerobic exercises use large muscles repeatedly, during which you maintain a designated exercise heart rate and sustain an even pace for many minutes. This submaximal, comfortable and steady pace allows improved circulation to the working muscles but is not so strenuous that it produces undue fatigue and early exhaustion.

Medical centers, community hospitals and private organizations throughout the country are currently offering medically supervised exercise programs for the general public as well as for rehabilitation of cardiac patients, and many YMCAs, YWCAs and other athletic clubs are now providing jumping-rebounding classes for their patrons. Of course, jumping in your own home provides many special benefits, but regardless of where you exercise, the approach usually involves a gradual, progressive build-up of jumping that reduces the possibility of muscle or joint injury and, most importantly, reduces or eliminates undue strain on the heart.

WHAT CAN YOU EXPECT FROM A JUMPING PROGRAM?

For the heart, plenty. Following the exercise program outlined in Chapter 10 should provide the cardiovascular benefits found in other aerobic activities. Just as with running, swimming or biking, jumping will increase the strength and size of the left ventricle of the heart, the chamber that pumps blood to the body; increase the blood output during each heartbeat; increase the diameter of the arteries of the heart; and increase the number of latent arteries used for distributing blood to the heart and the rest of the body.

It will also increase the total blood volume and the total amount of oxygen-carrying hemoglobin in the blood, beneficially slow the heart rate and decrease the amount of oxygen needed by the heart both at rest and during exercise. All of this adds up to one thing, a much fitter body and heart able to do more with less effort.

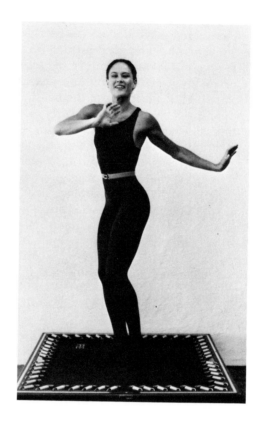

For body fat, you can expect benefits depending on how much you are willing to put into your jumping. You can burn off between 5 and 12 calories per minute, and if you exercise on a daily basis, that represents about 30 pounds of fat per year. Not only does the fat go off, but the muscle size and tone increase so that you get a much better-looking body as well.

The muscles will become stronger, firmer and larger, increase their efficiency in using oxygen and be more resistant to fatigue. And jumping will improve your agility, coordination and speed.

In addition, you can help strengthen the small muscles of the feet and reduce pain in the arches. Flat feet are often improved with the use of jumping, particularly when you jump barefoot. As you exercise you will lose weight and, as a result, there will be less stress on the arches and joints of the feet, ankles and knees. The human foot is very intricate and has about 26 separate bones. When your feet are abused by carrying extra weight, they will hurt.

And as for your head and psyche, it appears that exercising for extended periods of time can reduce stress and anxiety by reducing certain chemical messengers produced in our bodies which are responsible for that "up-tight" feeling.

IS THIS ONLY FOR ATHLETES?

Jumping is not for everyone. Still, we have found that jumping on good rebounding equipment is effective in improving the symptoms of over 80 percent of the patients reporting to our rehabilitation lab. Rebounding exercises have been used by both sexes of all ages as well as by individuals who have special orthopedic problems, such as mild arthritis, nondegenerative or nontraumatic low back pain syndrome, cardiac rehabilitation, pre- and post-knee and hip surgery, Osgood–Schlatter disease and osteochondritis; those suffering flat feet and arch strain, chronic shinsplints and certain neural disorders; and children with motor-perceptual disabilities. (See pages 189–192 for medical applications and supervision.)

Before using rebounders in our rehabilitation program, we decided to run a few tests. First we attached electronic shock-gauges to the legs, ankles and feet of our subjects so that we could determine the amount of impact to which their legs were subjected during exercise on grass, a hardwood floor, cement and rebounding equipment.

We found that jogging, jumping and skipping rope on rebounding equipment produced about one-third the impact that jogging on a treadmill or skipping rope on a floor would produce. In our laboratory, we also wanted to measure the amount of shock transmitted through the feet, ankles and legs while running at a $7\frac{1}{2}$-minute-per-mile pace (heart rate 150–165 beats per minute) and compare that with the shock transmitted at an equivalent to jogging in place on rebounding equipment at the identical 150–165-beat-per-minute heart rate.

In the study we found that during jogging the shock transmitted from the running surface of the treadmill up to the leg reached a force level of four to six times the body weight. While similarly exercising at the same heart rate on the rebounding equipment the force was reduced to a maximum of 1.7 to 2.2 times the body weight. Both of these experiments showed that rebounding exercise actually produces less leg trauma than walking, jogging or skipping rope on regular surfaces.

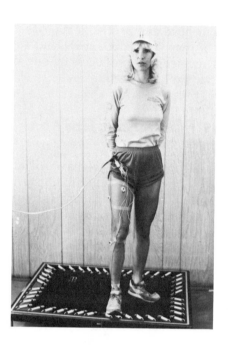

In a similar study conducted by Dr. A.U. Daniels, Adjunct Professor of Material Science and Engineering, and Orthopedic Surgery at the University of Utah, a rough comparison was made between the impact load transmitted on the aerobic springing gear versus the impact-load time factor for running on a board track. His study showed that the maximum impact experienced during exercise on rebounding equipment was only about 85 percent of that experienced during similar exercise on a board track.

In another study conducted in our laboratory, exercise was conducted on a treadmill, a stationary bike and on rebounding equipment. Seventy overweight women exercised five days per week at a heart rate of 150–175 beats per minute for about 40 minutes each day. The results showed that after ten weeks significant improvements in fitness and reductions in body fat were observed. The women were able to burn off calories at a rate of 8 to 12 per minute, resulting in a loss of between 9 and 15 pounds of body fat.

These studies showed that jumping was an effective exercise producing gains in fitness and reducing body fat, but causing less force

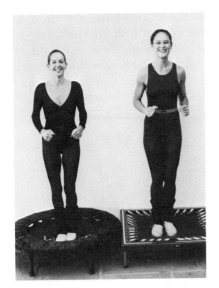
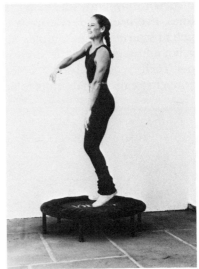

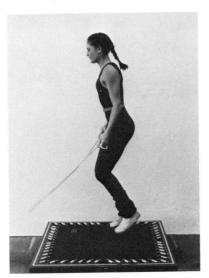

and trauma on the legs. A further look at this study showed that nearly half of those running on the treadmill sustained some type of foot, ankle or knee injury, while none of the women exercising on rebounding equipment experienced any significant pain, injury or discomfort.

From the medical point of view, rebounding equipment is not like the full-size trampoline, which specializes in high-flying bounces incorporating flips, turns and twists. Before using full-size trampolines, I've been told, one must receive special training from a competent instructor and employ stringent safety protocol. Jumping on rebounding gear is safer because stunts and acrobatic routines are not performed. Those who feel they may incur problems while bouncing can use side rails to add to stability and balance.

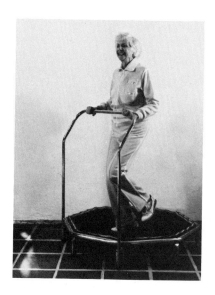
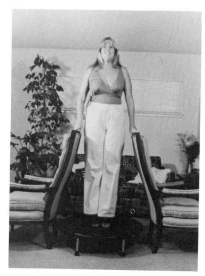

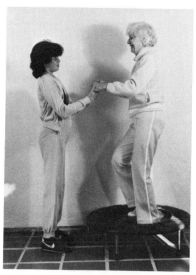

2

The Long-Range Benefits of Exercise

Although you probably look and feel good, beneath that apparent good health, and regardless of your age or sex, you could be building up a future case for coronary heart disease. We studied the health status of 60 entering freshmen at UCSD and followed those freshmen until their graduation four to five years later. Of the 60 incoming male and female freshmen, 80 percent were found to have two or more major coronary heart disease risk factors. These were 18- and 19-year-old American youths!

The major risk factors included high resting heart rate, elevated blood pressure, low physical fitness, high levels of anxiety, high levels of blood lipids, including cholesterol, inadequate nutrition, obesity, cigarette smoking, diabetes and adverse hereditary factors (for your risk factors, see Chapter 4).

Although nothing can be done about age, sex or heredity, we wanted to determine if during four years of college the other risk factors could be affected. To answer the question, half of the 60 students were put on a mandatory exercise program and the others were given a free choice of whether to exercise or not. The students on the exercise program were coerced, chided, and threatened into exercising on a near-daily basis. In fact, I personally spent at least two to three days each week participating in the exercise program with the students.

Those students who remained in college were tested again during their senior year and found to have significant changes in their heart disease risk factors. The students in the exercise program showed significant improvements in resting heart rate and physical fitness; they had less body fat and lower anxiety scores, and their blood pressure and blood lipid scores did not increase over the years. Students who exercised daily soon gave up the habit of smoking and didn't resume it during their four years of college.

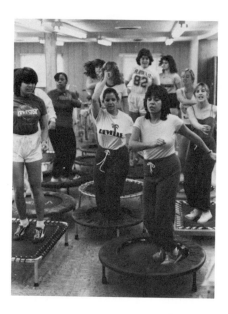

The students in the nonexercising group showed significant increases in resting heart rate and body fat, decreased physical fitness and increased anxiety scores. Extrapolating the blood pressure readings in this group, it was found that, by age 44, the male students would have blood pressures of 140/90 mmHg, the typical readings for middle-aged Americans, which result in a three-fold increase in the risk of developing coronary heart disease.

In the nonexercise group, the anxiety level nearly doubled between the freshman and senior years. Anxiety and depression accelerate the production of hormones called catecholamines. These hormones are secreted into the blood system, causing the heart rate and blood pressure to increase above normal. A well-conditioned person produces less of these stress hormones in the first place, and during exercise these hormones increase initially but then are dissipated after the exercise session.

Exercise stimulates the body's production of two other interesting chemicals: serotonin, a muscle relaxant similar in chemical structure to tranquilizers; and beta-endorphin, a morphinelike substance that produces the feeling of relaxation and enhanced mental attitude.

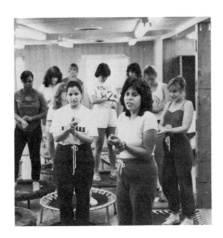

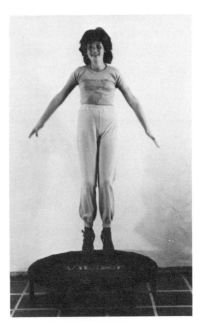

To get back to our study, those entering freshmen who smoked cigarettes averaged 14 cigarettes per day. Within six months the students in the exercising group had stopped using tobacco. The nonexercisers increased their consumption of cigarettes from 14 per day as freshmen to 28 per day as seniors.

Another interesting finding of this study was that the exercising group had a higher overall grade-point average than did the nonexercising group. The exercise group graduated with a 3.14 average (4.0 is equivalent to an *A*), and the nonexercising group had a grade-point average of 2.84. Furthermore, by the time the students graduated, only ten percent of the exercise group had two or more major coronary heart disease risk factors, while 90 percent of nonexercisers had two or more risk factors.

When you exercise you can expect to be healthier and more productive, reduce the number and severity of coronary heart disease risk factors, reduce anxiety and obesity, increase physical fitness and probably decrease or eliminate the use of tobacco.

3

Being in Shape

I'd like to share part of a letter we received from a worried female exerciser.

> I recently visited my gynecologist and he found that my heart rate was 52 beats per minute. He immediately transferred me to the emergency room for a resting electrocardiogram. After the ECG, the technician asked me if I was a jogger or an exerciser, and when I explained that I was, she said that slow pulse rates were expected in well-trained individuals. Why did my gynecologist become so upset, and is there something dangerous about having a slow heart rate?

Answering this question leads us into talking about the changes you can expect as you get into shape, either through jumping or through other forms of aerobic exercise. So, concerning our friend with the slow heart rate, if the slow heart rate (bradycardia) was the result of heart failure, as was suspected by her gynecologist, emergency treatment certainly would have been in order. Since she had been exercising for several months, however, it should have been expected that her heart rate would go from 70 to 80 beats per minute down to the 50s and 60s. In fact, many top male distance runners have resting heart rates in the middle 30s, and females, in the middle 40s. The problem was that this doctor hadn't seen enough patients who were in good shape to recognize that condition.

Exercise causes a response in the nervous system that reduces the heart rate. Low resting heart rates will continue as long as you continue to exercise.

YOUR BODY'S RESPONSE TO EXERCISE

Even when you merely think about exercise, you may get what is called an "anticipatory increase" in your heart rate because of the flow into the blood of certain body chemicals, the catecholamines, causing the heart to beat faster and increase the output of blood with each beat. When you start to exercise slowly, your heart rate and cardiac output will increase a bit, and they increase further as you exercise more vigorously.

As you continue to exercise, your breathing will get deeper and your heart rate will increase as the oxygen in the blood is transported to the working muscles in order to accommodate the increase in pace. From the moment exercise begins, there is an increase in the size of the arterioles (small arteries) of the working muscles, and there is an increase in the number of available capillaries (small vessels) used to transport blood through the body. As the arteries and capillaries widen, there is an actual decrease in the resistance to the blood flowing to the muscles. After exercise, there is often a beneficial drop in blood pressure that lasts for hours.

Blood Pressure and Exercise

Blood pressure is given as two numbers, a large number on top and a smaller number on the bottom. The large number (systolic pressure) is the pressure measured when your heart is contracting. It shows how hard your heart has to work to get blood out to the other cells of the body. The smaller number (diastolic pressure) is the pressure in your circulatory system when your heart relaxes. It's the resting, or "back," pressure of the system. The lower your systolic and diastolic pressures are (within reason), the less wear and tear there is on your heart and other organs. During exercise the systolic blood pressure tends to increase in proportion to the amount of work performed. For example, in the resting position, your systolic blood pressure may be 120 to 130 mmHg.*

During exercise of low intensity, blood pressure may increase up to 150 mmHg. At vigorous levels of exercise it may go to 180 mmHg,

---

*Doctors measure blood pressure by comparing it to the pressure exerted by a column of mercury in a glass tube. Since they measure the height of the mercury in millimeters (mm), and since the chemist's symbol for mercury is Hg, blood pressure is usually expressed as millimeters of mercury, or mmHg.

and at extremely intense levels it may go up to 200 or more mmHg. This high blood pressure during exercise is considered normal, and some researchers believe it may actually be beneficial in controlling hypertension (high blood pressure).

During exercise, the diastolic pressure may increase or decrease, depending on you as an individual. Resting diastolic pressure may be 70 to 80 mmHg. While it is slightly more common for the diastolic blood pressure to increase somewhat as the intensity of work increases, it is also very common for the diastolic blood pressure to fall to between 60 and 70 mmHg immediately after the end of the exercise.

Will Exercise Prolong Life?

While it is true that regular vigorous exercise reduces the statistical chances of heart disease, no one as yet has given absolute proof that it will promote longer life. But more and more doctors are running these days, and when the medical profession quietly picks up the practice, you know something is going on. (Three years ago a jogger would have been quite surprised to see more than one or two other joggers on the path. Today, the parks are crowded with joggers, and sales of exercise bicycles and rebounding equipment are at an all-time high. Additionally, large corporations are providing space and time for their executives and employees to participate in regular fitness programs.) And physicians are prescribing vigorous exercise for their patients because they feel it may help prevent heart disease, and they are prescribing exercise for their postcoronary patients as well.

How About Over-Fat Bodies?

Losing body fat is the result of combining regular vigorous exercise with reasonable nutrition. Studies conducted in our laboratory indicate that jumping for 30 to 40 minutes per day for five days a week for ten weeks will provide a substantial loss in body weight of about 4 to 10 pounds.

Greater improvements were seen in those same individuals after increasing their exercise time to 60 minutes a day, or an equivalent of jogging 4 to 6 miles. This equals a burn-off of about 500 calories per day. When jumping is combined with a reduction in unnecessary food of about 300 calories per day, a deficit of 800 calories is produced. This would represent a total loss of body fat of nearly 1.2 pounds per week, which equals 5 pounds a month or over 60 pounds a year.

Regular vigorous exercise not only reduces the amount of body fat but also reduces the amount of food eaten. Several studies have shown that by simply participating in daily vigorous exercise, you lessen the hunger sensation and reduce the amount of food you eat.

CORONARY HEART DISEASE PREVENTION

Coronary artery disease refers to the collection of cholesterol on the inner lining of the arteries that supply blood to the heart. Cholesterol is a fatty material that is carried in the blood. This process of clogging the arteries, known as atherosclerosis, occurs in many of the arteries of the body, and is accelerated when you use salt in the diet, eat saturated-fat foods (fatty meats and full-fat dairy products), smoke tobacco, are overweight, have high blood pressure and do not exercise regularly. Atherosclerosis can lead to symptoms of chest pain and, in many cases, to an actual heart attack.

Almost all experts agree that elevated blood pressure, cigarette smoking, high cholesterol levels and a lack of exercise are the major culprits in the development of this insidious disease. Evidence is starting to appear that reducing or eliminating these risk factors reverses this trend toward heart attack and premature death.

The question of how much exercise is required to protect against heart disease is not easily answered. Dr. Ralph Paffenbarger studied this question at the University of California at Berkeley, and he believes that you must engage in rather vigorous, frequent exercise in order to benefit, and that lighter exercise is not as effective in reducing heart disease. Paffenbarger claims that it is impossible to prove that exercise actually decreases heart attacks. However, people who participate in strenuous activities tend not to have heart disease. In contrast, those who participate in casual sports, such as golf, bowling, softball, baseball, volleyball and doubles tennis, tend to have a greater risk of heart disease.

THE HIDDEN BENEFITS OF EXERCISE

Impressive as the benefits of exercise listed in this chapter are, they may only scratch the surface. Every time those of us who study exercise take another look at its effects, we find that a person in good shape has all sorts of advantages over his or her sedentary friends.

To pick some examples, some of our still unfinished studies show that people's sex lives improve, and not just because they look more attractive but because their new fitness extends into the area of their sexual responses. We're doing more research now to see how to maximize that effect.

Another unexpected benefit of jumping is its effect on the bags under people's eyes. Many movie stars are characterized by large and interesting pouches underneath their eyes. In some cases these pouches are really the accumulation of fat cells. As an individual becomes more obese, the fat cells enlarge and fluid tends to accumulate in these areas. This gives the fullness that eventually may cause the excess skin to bag and sag. These can be reduced surgically, but clinical observations tell us that those who commence and adhere to vigorous exercise will probably reduce the size of these fat pads and reduce the fluid retention in the area.

We have researched the subject and have been unable to find very much information, but if you are experiencing unwanted bags under your eyes, take a photograph of your face now, see your physician about proceeding with an exercise program and, with his/her approval, proceed with the exercise program described in this book. Take another picture in about three months and don't be amazed if those bags look "unpacked." This has happened to several people in our jumping program.

4

Your Risk Factor Profile

Ready to determine your health status? Most of us see our physicians once a year or so—doctors are usually concerned with finding disease and not with assessing health. Often they don't have time to explain things at length.

As explained in Chapter 2, there are risk factors for coronary heart disease. By taking a simple test, you can approximate your health status. The results won't be as accurate or revealing as a physical examination by your doctor, but we've found that our test gives a surprisingly accurate health profile to symptom-free people who take it.

This chapter has three parts. The first is a Risk Factor Questionnaire, which you will take like any other test (and be honest with yourself in answering the questions). The second is a Health Profile on which you will record your scores from the questionnaire and graphically depict your health status. In the third part, we'll discuss the questionnaire, section by section, and tell you why you got the score you did and how you can improve it. (Remember, this chapter isn't here to scare you. It's here to show where you could use some improvements in your life-style, and later in the book we'll show you how to make those improvements.)

So let's get on with the questionnaire by circling the single number that answers each question most accurately. Next, add the numbers that have been circled and record the total for each section in the designated box. Sections E and F have subsections. Be sure to score the subsections and then add up the scores and put them in the appropriate box. After completing the questionnaire, enter the ten scores on your health profile and draw a line beneath the score as seen in the example (page 33).

RISK FACTOR PROFILE

(A) + (B) + (C) TOTAL SCORE _____

(A) AGE

(A) SCORE _____

MALE		FEMALE	
72 and over	3	78 and over	3
71–68	0	78–75	2
67–64	1	74–70	1
63–61	2	69–66	0
60–57	3	65–60	2
56–54	4	59–54	4
53–49	5	53–46	6
48–44	6	45–38	7
43–40	7	37–30	8
39–35	8	29–21	9
34–21	9	20 and under	10
20 and under	10		

(B) GENDER

(B) SCORE _____

MALE	
stocky build, bald	−1
stocky build	0
average build	2
slight build	3

FEMALE	
any age, postmenopause	5
age 55 or over, premenopause	7
age 54–50	8
age 48–36	9
age 35 and under	10

(C) FAMILY HISTORY

(C) SCORE _____

I have the following number of family members (parents, brothers, sisters and grandparents) who had heart disease or stroke which occurred between the indicated ages.

ONE FAMILY MEMBER

age 30 or less	−8
age 31–40	−2
age 41–50	0
age 51–55	1
age 56–60	2
age 61–65	3
age 66–70	4
age 70 or over	7
none	10

If parents are not known circle 5.

TWO OR MORE FAMILY MEMBERS

age 30 or less	−12
age 31–40	−8
age 41–50	−4
age 51–60	−2
age 61–70	0
age 71–75	1
age 75 or over	5

(D) BREATHING POLLUTION
PULMONARY STATUS

(D) SCORE _____

Never smoked anything	10
Smoked cigarettes or marijuana but quit:	
more than 15 years ago	9
11–15 years ago	8
6–10 years ago	7
1–5 years ago	6
less than 1 year ago	3
Currently smoke:	
1 marijuana cigarette/week or 1–5 cigarettes/day	−3
pipe or cigar or cigarettes but do not intentionally inhale	−4
2 marijuana cigarettes/week or 6–11 cigarettes/day	−5
3–6 marijuana cigarettes/week or 12–19 cigarettes/day	−8
1 marijuana cigarette/day or 1 pack cigarettes/day	−10
2 marijuana cigarettes/day plus 10 or more cigarettes/day	−12
3 or more marijuana cigarettes/day or 3 or more packs cigarettes/day	−15
I have worked in a smoky office for:	
more than 20 years	−3
10–20 years	−2
I have lived with smokers for:	
more than 20 years	−3
10–20 years	−2
I have lived in a smoggy area such as Los Angeles for:	
10 years or more	−2
1–9 years	−1
I have or had emphysema	−3

(E) FOOD AND NUTRITION

(E) TOTAL SCORE _____

(E-1)

(E-1) SCORE _____

I feel I overeat:
usually	0
occasionally	1
rarely	3

I skip meals:
at least once a day	0
3–5 per week	1
rarely	3

I salt my food or eat salty foods:
often	0
occasionally	1
rarely	3

(E-2)

(E-2) SCORE _____

My daily soft drink (8 oz cola) consumption is:
3 or more	0
1 or 2	1
none	3

My daily tea consumption is:
5 or more cups	0
3 or 4 cups	1
2 cups or less	2
noncaffeine herbal tea	3

My daily coffee consumption is:
4 or more cups	0
2 or 3 cups	1
decaffeinated	2
1 cup or less	3

(E-3)

My refined sugar, honey and sweet food consumption is:

    average or above 0

    less than average 1

    very low 3

Most drinks contain 1–1.5 oz of alcohol.

My daily alcohol consumption is:

    3 or more drinks 0

    2 drinks 2

    1 drink 3

    none 1

For dessert I usually eat:

    pie or cake, cookies, ice cream, cheese cake, etc 0

    gelatin dessert, puddings, canned fruits 1

    fresh fruits 3

For snacks I usually eat:

    candy, pastry or ice cream 0

    processed foods or canned fruits 1

    fresh fruits, vegetables, and whole grain items 3

(E-4)

My daily roughage intake consists of:

    normal diet 0

    extra salad and raw vegetables 1

    bran, pectin or metamucil once or twice a day 3

My bread and / or cereal consists of:

    white bread and / or regular boxed sweetened cereals 0

    whole grain breads and / or whole grain cereals 3

(E-5)

My dairy products consist of:

whole milk/cream products (most cheeses) or imitation dairy
products 0

low-fat dairy products 1

skim milk (non-fat) dairy products, low-fat cheeses 3

My total daily meat and cheese consumption is:

8 oz or more 0

6 oz 1

4–5 oz 2

3 oz or less 3

I use:

lard or generous amounts of oils, nuts, vegetable shortening, but-
ter or margarine 0

limited amounts of oils, nuts, butter, vegetable shortening or
margarine 1

I rarely use oils, nuts, butter or margarine 3

My total weekly egg consumption is:

9 or more 0

6–8 1

5 or less 3

My diet generally includes:

meats (pork, beef, duck, liver, organ meats, hamburger,
steak) 0

meats (lean beef, veal, chicken, turkey and fish cooked with
skin) 1

lean meats (fish, chicken, veal, turkey cooked without skin); no
meat at all or meat substitutes: beans, rice, etc 3

(F) PERSONALITY

(F) TOTAL SCORE _____

(F-1)

(F-1) SCORE _____

I have several projects going on at one time:

usually	0
occasionally	1
rarely	3

I would describe myself as:

competitive/hard driving	0
moderately competitive	1
not competitive	3

I become irritated when kept waiting:

usually	0
occasionally	1
rarely	3

I make important decisions:

often	0
occasionally	1
seldom	3

I try to accomplish a great deal each day:

almost always	0
frequently	1
occasionally	2
rarely	4

In my work, success is:

very important	0
moderately important	1
not important	3

I have important deadlines:

often	0
occasionally	1
rarely	3

People disappoint me:

often	0
occasionally	1
rarely	3

(F-2)

(F-2)SCORE _____

I feel a lump in the pit of my stomach:
    almost always 0
    frequently 1
    occasionally 3
    rarely 4
I am anxious / nervous:
    often 0
    occasionally 1
    seldom 3
I have disturbed sleep:
    often 0
    occasionally 1
    seldom 3

(F-3)

(F-3)SCORE _____

When confronted with a situation that bothers or angers me:
    I keep it to myself 0
    I may or may not say something 1
    I always say something about it 3
I have spells of the blues:
    often 0
    occasionally 1
    seldom 3
I laugh heartily:
    seldom 0
    occasionally 1
    frequently 3

(F-4)

I got along with my parents:

    not well at all 0

    fairly well 1

    beautifully 3

I am sexually frustrated or dissatisfied:

    often 0

    occasionally 1

    rarely 3

Criticism or scolding bothers me:

    greatly 0

    moderately 1

    hardly at all 3

I am secretive:

    greatly 0

    moderately 1

    hardly at all 3

(G)EXERCISE, OCCUPATION, RECREATION

My exercise/recreation consists of:

    little or no exercise 0

    walking program 3 or more days/week 1

    easy to moderate exercise 3 or more days/week 2

    fairly vigorous exercise in exercise attire 3–4 days/week 7

    heavy exercise in exercise attire 5–7 days/week 15

My occupational activities consist of:

    mostly mental activity with little or no manual labor 0

    combination of mental and manual labor 2

    mostly manual labor; I perspire from my work 4

(H)PAST AND PRESENT HEALTH STATUS

(H)SCORE _____

Have had a heart attack or heart disease .... −10
Have not had a heart attack or heart disease but have had heart or
chest pain (angina) when I exercise .... −5
Have or have had:
    diabetes (receiving insulin) .... −5
    kidney disorders .... −3
    thyroid conditions .... −3
    gout .... −3

(I)BLOOD PRESSURE

(I)TOTAL SCORE _____

If no technician is available to determine your body fat and blood pressure,
complete to your best ability. If not known, circle 5 for (I-1) and (I-2).

SYSTOLIC BLOOD PRESSURE (I-1)SCORE _____

MEN	WOMEN Premenopause	WOMEN Postmenopause	SCORE
184	177	180	−5
164	157	160	−3
154	147	150	−2
144	137	140	0
139	132	135	4
134	127	130	5
129	122	125	6
125	119	121	7
122	116	118	8
118	113	115	9
113	108	110	10

DIASTOLIC **BLOOD PRESSURE (I-2) SCORE** _____

MEN	WOMEN Premenopause	WOMEN Postmenopause	SCORE
99	99	99	−5
97	95	96	−3
95	90	93	−2
92	88	90	0
88	86	88	2
86	83	84	5
82	78	80	6
76	73	75	7
73	68	70	8
68	66	68	9
65	63	65	10

(J) BODY FAT

(J) TOTAL SCORE_____

TABLE I Use this table only if percent body fat has been measured by the method on pages 41−46.

Percent Body Fat

MALE		FEMALE	
30 and over	0	35 and over	0
29−28	1	34−32	1
27−25	2	31−29	2
24−22	3	28−27	3
21−20	4	26−25	4
19−18	5	24−23	5
17−16	6	22−21	6
15−14	7	20−19	7
13−12	8	18−17	8
11	9	16−15	9
10 and under	10	14 and under	10

TABLE II Use this table only if percent body fat has not been measured. Considering what you think to be your most desirable weight, you are presently:

76 or more lbs over	−5
51–75 lbs over	0
41–50 lbs over	1
31–40 lbs over	2
21–30 lbs over	3
16–20 lbs over	4
11–15 lbs over	5
7–10 lbs over	6
4–6 lbs over	7
1–3 lbs over	8
at or below that weight	10

SCORING SHEET

Enter total points from sections:

(A) + (B) + (C)	_____	Age, Gender, Family History
(D)	_____	Pulmonary
(E)	_____	Nutrition
(F)	_____	Personality, Stress
(G)	_____	Exercise / Recreation, Occupation
(H)	_____	Past / Present Health
(I)	_____	Blood Pressure
(J)	_____	Percent Body Fat
	_____	**TOTAL SCORE**

Now, write your scores on the "Health Profile."

SUMMARY SCALE:

Exceptionally low risk	over 130
Excellent, very low risk	111–129
Very good, low risk	100–110
Satisfactory, low risk	90–99
Average risk	80–89
Poor risk	70–79
Dangerous risk	60–69
Extremely dangerous risk	below 60

Two of the measurements on your Health Profile, percent body fat and VO$_2$ max (fitness), will be explained in Chapters 5 and 6. After you've read those chapters, you'll know how to estimate those values and you can come back and enter your own measurements for VO$_2$ max and percent body fat to complete the Health Profile.

Remember, your Health Profile is not an absolute measure of your health because it does not cover every health item. However, it will allow you to estimate your statistical chance of future disease, heart attack or stroke.

Now that you have completed your own Health Profile, what does it mean? Well, each health item plays a significant role in your total health plan.

Let's look at your profile for a moment. Compare it to the example on page 33. Are most of your scores below average? If so, you probably need to make some very specific changes. If some of your scores are high, some are low, and some are right on the average, you might want to consider taking steps to bolster the areas in which you have scored poorly. It's our hope that you will be able to follow the suggestions and eventually get all your scores up above the average. It wasn't that long ago, in 1969, in fact, that I scored below average on every item on the profile; I was a fat waddler just struggling along and not exercising. I made changes in my life that worked, and I'd like to share with you personal methods and suggestions that have worked on well over 10,000 people during the last 14 years.

Age (A), Gender (B) and Family History (C)

As you know, the older we get, the more we wear out, and each year we tend to get a little more susceptible to health problems. As far as aging goes, we do know that there are three major ways you can reduce the aging process. The first, of course, is to eat properly and keep your body thin; the second is to exercise four to five days per week; and, finally, we know that smoking accelerates the aging process, causes excess wrinkles in the skin and shortens one's life. Not a very good trade-off.

The next item, gender, is very simple. Women tend to live longer than men by two to three years and some studies figure an additional eight years of longevity. Researchers believe that testosterone (the male hormone) may contribute to the heart disease that is so frequently found in males. Recently, some evidence has been found that males who have a stocky build and are bald may be especially susceptible.

The final item in this section is concerned with hereditary factors (the characteristics you inherit from your parents). Like age and gender, heredity cannot be changed. You just don't get the opportunity to select your parents.

If you have blood relatives who've had heart disease, stroke, or diabetes, it doesn't mean that you are going to acquire those diseases. However, it increases your statistical chance, and if you happen to score below the average in this section, you might want to take special care to make life-style changes that will get your scores as high as possible in the sections you *can* influence.

Breathing, Pollution and Smoking Habits (D)

If you smoke tobacco, you're at a disadvantage. The following information is kind of interesting, but if you're a smoker and not that interested, why don't you just skip this section for now. For those who *are* interested, I'll share some bits of information we've collected.

In a review of over 45,000 studies on tobacco and tobacco use, we could not find one article that showed that the use of tobacco enhances health. In fact, tobacco use increases the user's chance of having heart disease by 200 to 300 percent, and there is a ten-fold increase in the chance of developing cancer. For women, smoking and drinking coffee increase the chance of breast cancer by 6,000 percent! Not only does smoking impair hearing, eyesight, manual dexterity and reflexes, it causes significant increases in resting heart rate and in bronchial constriction (which results in increased breathing resistance), and, interestingly, causes a hand tremor in young men, women, and children that would be expected in an 80-year-old person.

All cigarette smokers have what are called pre-cancer cells in their lungs. The pre-cancer cells may or may not develop into active cancer cells, but it takes over two years of not smoking for those cells to return back to normal, functioning cells.

Finally, the number, width and depth of wrinkles in 40-year-old women smokers are the same as those found in 60-year-old non-smokers. Studies from Europe show that inhaling tobacco smoke reduces testosterone levels, which causes reduced sex drive in males, especially those 40 years of age or older.

While smokers agree that smoking is not good for their health, a recent study conducted in our laboratory and reported in the *New England Journal of Medicine* showed that nonsmokers living or working with smokers develop between 5 and 15 percent lung impairment. Researcher Dr. Tager, in a Harvard University study (1980), found similar damage in children whose parents smoked.

The best advice for your heart, lungs, nervous system and skin, therefore, is to stay away from tobacco smoke.

HEALTH PROFILE*

Category	Excellent	Very good	Good	Satisfactory	Average	Unsatisfactory	Very poor	Extremely poor
Incidence of CHD ♀+	0.1	0.2	0.4	0.7	1.0	2.8	4.6	
Incidence of CHD ♂→	0.1	0.3	0.5	1.0	2.0	8.0	12.0	24.0
Percentile	90	80	70	60	50	40	30	20
TOTAL SCORE	Over 130	110–129	100–109	90–99	80–89	70–79	60–69	Under 60
(J) Percent Body Fat	10	8	7	6	5	4	3	2
(I) Blood Pressure	20	17	15	12	5	0	-2	-6
(H) Health Status	0	0	0	-3	-6	-8	-15	-20
(G) Exercise/Occupation and VO_2 max	19	15	11	8	6	5	4	3
(F) Personality — Sensitivity/Withdrawal/Shyness (4)	12	10	9	7	5	4	3	2
(F) Personality — Depression (3)	9	7	5	4	3	2	1	0
(F) Personality — Anxiety (2)	10	9	8	6	5	3	1	0
(F) Personality — Type A (1)	25	19	13	10	8	6	4	2
(E) Nutrition — Fats in Diet (5)	15	11	9	7	5	4	3	2
(E) Nutrition — Roughage in Diet (4)	6	6	5	4	3	2	1	0
(E) Nutrition — Sugar Intake (3)	12	10	8	6	5	4	3	2
(E) Nutrition — Caffeine Intake (2)	9	7	5	4	3	2	1	0
(E) Nutrition — Eating Habits (1)	9	8	7	6	5	4	3	2
(D) Lungs/Breathing	10	7	6	3	0	-3	-12	-18
(A)(B)(C) Age—Gender—Heredity	30	21	18	14	12	10	8	6

⌐ Record your scores in this row

* Reprinted with permission from Institute for Health Management, 2310 Mason St., San Francisco, CA 94133.

SAMPLE HEALTH PROFILE

Factor	Your Score	Excellent	Very good	Good	Satisfactory	Average	Unsatisfactory	Very poor	Extremely poor
Incidence of CHD ♀		0.1	0.2	0.4	0.7	1.0	2.8	4.6	
Incidence of CHD ♂		0.1	0.3	0.5	1.0	2.0	8.0	12.0	24.0
Percentile		90	80	70	60	50	40	30	20
DESCRIPTION		Excellent	Very good	Good	Satisfactory	Average	Unsatisfactory	Very poor	Extremely poor
TOTAL SCORE	68	Over 130	110–129	100–109	90–99	80–89	70–79	60–69	Under 60
(J) Percent Body Fat	5	10	8	7	6	5	4	3	2
(I) Blood Pressure	8	20	17	15	12	5	0	-2	-6
(H) Health Status	-3	0	0	0	-3	-6	-9	-15	-20
(G) Exercise / Occupation and VO₂ max	3	19	15	11	8	6	5	4	3
(F) Personality — Sensitivity / Withdrawal / Shyness [4]	11	12	10	9	7	5	4	3	2
(F) Personality — Depression [3]	8	9	7	5	4	3	2	1	0
(F) Personality — Anxiety [2]	3	10	9	8	6	5	3	1	0
(F) Personality — Type A [1]	4	25	19	13	10	8	6	4	2
(E) Nutrition — Fats in Diet [5]	7	15	11	9	7	5	4	3	2
(E) Nutrition — Roughage in Diet [4]	0	6	6	5	4	3	2	1	0
(E) Nutrition — Sugar Intake [3]	2	12	10	8	6	5	4	3	2
(E) Nutrition — Caffeine Intake [2]	9	9	7	5	4	3	2	1	0
(E) Nutrition — Eating Habits [1]	2	9	8	7	6	5	4	3	2
(D) Lungs / Breathing	-3	10	7	6	3	0	-3	-12	-18
(A)(B)(C) Age—Gender—Heredity	12	30	21	18	14	12	10	8	6

Record your scores in this row

Food and Diet (E)

A glance at this section shows that not just how much we eat but also what we eat and the way we eat it affects our risk factor profile. That's good news, because we *can* control our eating. We may not be able to change parents or alter our personalities, but there's no excuse for not eating smarter, which often means eating a little less.

All the advice on how to eat well—and it's the best advice from the best laboratories in the country—is collected and expanded in Chapter 12. You can either skip to it right now, or you can save it for later when we show you new eating habits for a thinner you. For your convenience, the recommendations in Chapter 12 are condensed here.

ADVICE FOR NEW EATING HABITS

(E) NUTRITION

(E-1) Overeating is caused by:

—skipping meals
—dieting for rapid weight loss
—gluttony
—not exercising
—excessive sugar and alcohol

So . . .
—don't overload your plate
—don't go back for seconds
—don't eat off others' plates after you are finished
—don't order, buy and eat high-fat foods
—don't eat products containing sugar—eat fresh fruit
—don't go on crazy diets—eat three reasonable meals a day
—don't take more than 1–2 drinks of alcohol a day

Skipping meals:
—makes you an overeater later that day
—makes you nervous, less productive, irritable, constantly hungry and unhappy

So . . . eat a little less each meal, but never skip a meal

Salt:
Causes high blood pressure and increases risk of CHD, stroke and kidney dysfunction.

So . . . buy and eat less salted potato chips, corn chips, pickles, sauerkraut, and processed meats. At home, replace salt in shaker with a salt substitute. Read the labels on boxed, frozen or canned foods, and avoid if salt or sodium is mentioned. If you must, lightly salt meat and eggs, nothing more.

(E-2) Caffeine

Is found in coffee (100–150 mg), tea (70 mg), chocolate (30–50 mg), cola drinks (10–30 mg). Is related to breast cancer and may cause nervousness, tension, feelings of insecurity, lack of interest and nervous disorders. Avoid by drinking non-caffeine drinks such as herbal tea, fruit juice and water. Avoid consuming more than 150 mg of caffeine a day.

(E-3) Sugar

—causes body fat
—may be related to hypoglycemia and diabetes
—usually causes nervousness
—may strip Vitamin B from the nervous system and leave it less stable

Don't sprinkle sugar on your food and read the labels on processed foods. Avoid if sugar is mentioned among the first four items.

Honey, brown sugar, and molasses are about the same as sugar.

When you want sweet food, eat fresh fruit. Careful, most canned and frozen fruit have sugar added.

(E-4) Roughage

90 percent of U.S. diets are low in roughage, containing only 1–2 grams per day. Low roughage diets often cause hemorrhoids, diverticulitis and cancer of the colon.

You need 10 grams of roughage a day. Add one or two tablespoons of unprocessed bran to diet early in the day. Moisten before eating. Eat an apple a day for pectin . . . it lowers your cholesterol.

(E-5) Fats

Among all the calories you eat each day, 40 percent are from fats, most of them saturated fats. Saturated fats are found in cheese, hamburger, bacon, sausage, prime rib, steak and foods fried in animal fat or coconut oils.

Eating fats causes your body to be fat, elevates your blood pressure, cholesterol and other lipids, and increases your chances of developing CHD, diabetes and cancer.

In the market:
−select low-fat and non-fat dairy products
−go easy on all oils, butter and cream products
−buy lean meats, chicken, turkey, veal, fish and seafoods (remove all skin and fat before cooking)
−limit your total intake of cheese and meat to 3−4 oz per day
−try one or two days a week with vegetarian diets

Personality (F)

We find that personality characteristics are difficult to change after puberty, but there *are* several ways to deal with anxiety, stress, nervous tension, frustration, dissatisfaction and depression. Let's take a look.

Section F1 looks at the type-A personality. This is the overachiever possessed by a little demon that makes him or her a poor listener, anxious to get things started and finished, unsympathetic to others, highly productive and hard-driven. The type A seeks jobs that keep him or her under constant stress and the pressure of urgent deadlines, which provides an excuse for the frantic behavior so typical of this personality type.

The type A needs to understand that the stress is self-imposed, and should attempt to reduce stress in the occupation, avoid stressful situations whenever possible and learn to accept what cannot be changed.

The remaining portions of the personality section deal with depression, frustration, sensitivity and anxiety. Should your scores fall well below the average, we recommend that you consider seeking psychological counseling.

We now have evidence that chronic unresolved anxiety increases heart disease, ulcers and cancer. Anxiety also reduces the ability to concentrate, learn and produce. In general terms, daily vigorous exercise reduces the production of debilitating hormones and chemicals that are produced in response to stress, and increases the growth hormones and what we might term "healthy" hormones.

To further cope with stress, make sure that your nutrition includes an ample amount of Vitamin C, possibly two or three 500 mg pills each day as well as a multivitamin pill that contains adequate amounts of zinc and copper. Additionally, high-potency B-complex supplements have been effective in maintaining a more stable nervous system.

Finally, locate the stressful situations in your life, confront them straight on—one at a time—and attempt to resolve each problem. Don't take on too much at one time, and remember that professional counseling is often helpful.

Exercise, Occupation, Recreation (G)

Vigorous daily exercise may increase longevity or at least reduce the occurrence of heart disease and heart attacks. We feel certain that participating in vigorous exercise cuts in half the chance of incurring a *fatal* heart attack.

The types of exercise we would recommend are aerobic in nature: jogging, brisk walking, swimming, bicycling, cross-country skiing, rope skipping and, of course, jumping for joy. The exercise should be maintained four to seven days per week. If you follow the program outlined in Chapter 9, you will be able to increase the amount of time you exercise progressively, therefore reducing your body fat, and at the same time you will reduce your stress and anxiety. There is no shortcut to physical fitness, and recent claims that fitness can be achieved in 30 minutes per week are unproven and absurd.

As for your occupational activities, 95 percent of all Americans do not achieve fitness in their jobs. If you work at a job where you perspire vigorously for eight hours a day, and your heart rate is kept at a moderately high pace during most of that time, an exercise program will simply improve your present level of fitness. If, however, you are a typical American chained to a desk, tethered to a boss, or glued to the television, you definitely need between 30 and 60 minutes of exercise per day to keep your body thin, keep your anxiety down and reduce your chance of unnecessary future disease.

Health Status (H)

This section deals primarily with your present and past health status. It is included here to remind you to see your doctor and have a checkup if you receive a negative score in this category. Most of the items are related to coronary heart disease risk factors or to other disease states, and if they are unattended, they may develop into something more serious in future years.

Blood Pressure (I)

We all know that high blood pressure is dangerous. If you're like most of us, your blood pressure has quietly and insidiously increased over the years. But do you know that you can function effectively and yet be unaware that an insidious "silent killer" is lurking in your arteries.

I think a story might be appropriate here about one such person. She was an executive in her middle 40s, and she came to UCSD for an evaluation. She felt absolutely fine, but her blood pressure was 160/92 mmHg. Her physician felt that her blood pressure was not extensively elevated and that, although medication wasn't necessary, cutting down on salt and losing a little weight would be of benefit.

We consulted with her physician and together decided that a more aggressive preventive program should be ordered. She was put on a diet very low in saturated fats, and we eliminated salt, caffeine, nicotine and refined carbohydrates (sugar, honey, white-flour products). She enrolled in an exercise class at the YMCA and, in addition, started a vigorous daily jumping program. Within nine months she had lost two dress sizes, was significantly more productive in her business and had reduced her blood pressure to a respectable 127/85 mmHg. We're not sure which particular change contributed most to reducing her blood pressure, but we feel that all of the changes contributed in some significant degree to the overall success.

Body Fat (J)

We have found in our laboratory that over 80 percent of the women and 75 percent of the men we test have excess body fat. The amount of fat has ranged from just a few to over 260 pounds of excess body fat!

Excess body fat alone may not cause heart disease, but in combination with elevated blood sugar, elevated blood pressure and elevated lipids, or in combination with cigarette smoking, it does pose serious potential harm by contributing to heart disease, diabetes and cancer. Usually, overweight occurs in combination with one of the above abnormalities, and while it's difficult to become thin, our motto is "get thin and stay thin."

In most cases, being overweight is simply a case of eating a little too much and underexercising. In some cases, however, we have found that radical dieting and vigorous exercise do not produce the trim individual we had hoped for. This occurs more frequently in females, and while it does take longer to achieve success for these individuals, they must make additional sacrifices, especially in the field of exercise.

We have found that women who eat properly and exercise regularly and still do not lose weight are probably not exercising vigorously enough or long enough. These individuals must more than double their exercise participation to achieve a normal weight reduction. And, while we're on the subject, it has been a clinical observation that women must exercise 20 to 40 percent more or longer than men to achieve a proportional amount of body-fat loss. (More information on this appears on page 90.)

Swimmers attempting to lose body fat have more difficulty than those exercising on bicycles, joggers or jumpers. Apparently nature has provided us humans with a layer of fat cells that tend to stay full of lipids to act as insulation for swimming in cold water.

Remember, if you exercise about an hour a day, you burn around 300 to 600 calories, and if you cut 300 calories from your diet, that creates a caloric loss of at least 600 a day, or 3600 calories a week. Once again, 1 pound of fat equals 3500 calories. A 3500-calorie deficit each week would allow you to lose approximately 52 pounds of body fat by next year!

5

How Fat Is Your Body?

Everybody needs to know, so let's determine your percentage of body fat. You can keep it a secret if you want.

Between skin and muscle is a layer of fat cells. When you eat too much and don't exercise, those cells slowly, over the years, fill up with fat, become larger, and give your entire body a pudgy look. There are more fat cells around the thighs, hips, stomach and on the back of the upper arms than on other parts of the body. Unfortunately, women have many more fat cells than men, the cells are larger, and the result is that women naturally carry more body fat than men. Even within the same sex, people differ as to where their cells are located and how much fat collects in them.

We can determine how much fat your body is carrying by measuring the thickness of the fat at different locations. Remember it is not necessarily how much you weigh that counts, but how much fat is hiding beneath your skin. For example, several women began a program of proper nutrition and jumping 50 minutes daily for three months, and actually *gained* weight. They were disturbed because they had worked so conscientiously and still gained 3 to 5 pounds. Naturally, they wondered if the program was working.

We assured them that the program was working very well, and showed them that their percent body fat had dropped from 30 percent down to a more respectable 26 percent, a whopping 13-percent overall decrease in fat in only three months. Additionally, they had dropped one to two dress sizes—they had actually gained weight while their bodies had gotten smaller!

The reason is very simple. Their exercise program had built up their muscles to a normal size, while the fat cells had reduced back to their normal size. If you're interested in the mathematics, it goes like this: Initially the women weighed an average of 124 pounds, of which 13 pounds was excess fat. The three months of exercising burned an equivalent of 13 pounds of fat, but jumping also produced a 16-pound gain in lean and trim muscle. Since fat takes up more room than muscle, they actually shrank in size and gained in weight. Not a bad switch.

Similar results are seen in men. They gain in strength and muscle as they lose in belt size. In general, men should have about 12 to 17 percent body fat, with the optimum at 12 percent, and women, around 18 to 25 percent, with the optimum at about 22 percent.

Follow the instructions on the following pages to measure your percent body fat. After you have measured, you'll probably find that you are a bit overfat. Don't be discouraged; we have a plan for you. The plan is simple. We'll give you an eating program that you can live with, and an exercise program that's fun.

FOR WOMEN

OK, let's get out the tape measure and see how you measure up. The following steps will give you a fairly good idea about your level of fatness:

1. With a cloth tape, measure the girth of the right thigh approximately 1 inch below the crotch.
   Enter here: ____ in.

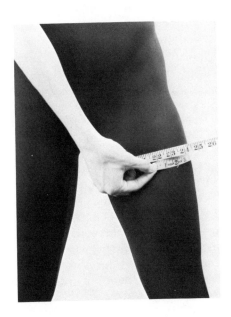

2. Measure the girth of the right biceps at the mid-muscle belly (the midpoint of the biceps). If you are alone, you can tape one end of the tape measure and gently pull it around for the measurement as shown below.

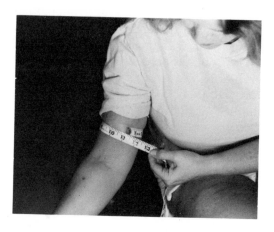

   Enter here: ____ in.
3. Add thigh and arm girth measurements.
   Enter total here: ____ in.
4. Locate the total of the two measurements on Table 5.1 for an estimate of your percent body fat. For example, if the sum of the two measurements equals 27 inches, your estimated body fat is 16 percent. If you measure 45 inches, your estimated body fat is 40 percent.
   Enter percent body fat here: ____ percent.

   Let's say the measurement came out as 24 percent body fat (female). Turn back to page 28, section J, and you'll see that you earn 5 points on your Health Profile. Enter your earned percent body fat score on page 28 under "Total Score." Next, enter the appropriate points on your Health Profile on page 32.
   I have found that most people know exactly what they should weigh. If I asked you how much you should weigh, your answer would most likely be within 5 pounds of your absolute ideal weight as determined by the most sophisticated methods measurement. After questioning 1580 women, the general consensus of what they should weigh is depicted in Table 5.2.
   If your percent body fat is a little higher than you're willing to settle for, be encouraged—we're going to show you how to take that fat off and keep it off.

TABLE 5.1. PERCENT BODY FAT* FOR WOMEN

Total Girths in Inches	Estimated Percent Body Fat	
25	12	Very lean
26	14	
27	16	
28	18	Lean
29	20	
30	22	
31	23	Good; leaner than average
32	24	
33	25	
34	26	Fair; a bit overfat but average
35	27	
35.5	28	
36	29	Overfat
37	30	
38	31	
39	32	You have put too much time into non-active business. Take care of yourself. You need to "Jump for Joy" regularly to reduce your level of fatness.
40	34	
41	35	
42	36	
43	37	
44	38	
45	40	
46	41	
47	42	
48	43	
49	44	
50	46	

*From thigh and upper arm girths.

TABLE 5.2. ANSWERS OF 1580 WOMEN TO "WHAT IS YOUR IDEAL WEIGHT?"

Height	Thin	Normal	Over-Fat
4′ 10″	96	105	127
5′ 0″	102	110	137
5′ 2″	106	116	145
5′ 4″	113	123	154
5′ 6″	120	130	160
5′ 8″	125	137	171
5′ 10″	131	144	180
6′ 0″	135	152	190
6′ 2″	141	160	199
6′ 4″	153	166	208

FOR MEN

This measuring technique should give you men a fairly accurate idea of your level of fatness.

   1. Use a cloth tape measure to determine the number of inches around your middle. Measure several times at the belly button.

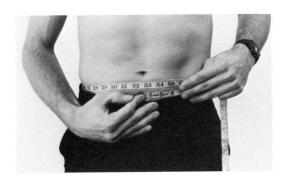

       Enter here: ____ in.
   2. Using an accurate scale, determine your body weight.
      Enter here: ____ in.
      Now go to Table 5.3, place a straight-edge ruler between the two scores and look at the middle line to read your percent body fat. For example, if you weigh 180 pounds and have a waist of 35 inches, your percent body fat is approximately 19 percent. If you have a 30-inch waist and weigh 145 pounds, you have approximately 10 percent body fat. Your ideal body fat is between 12 and 17 percent.
      Enter here: ____ percent.

Let's say that you measure 24 percent body fat using this method. Turn to page 28 (section J) and observe that you earn 5 points on the Health Profile. Enter your percent body fat on page 28, then enter your points in your Health Profile on page 32.

    I have found that most people know exactly what they should weigh. If I asked you how much you should weigh, your answer would most likely be within 5 pounds of your absolute ideal weight as determined by the most sophisticated methods measurement. After questioning 2470 men, the general consensus of what they should weigh is depicted in Table 5.4.

TABLE 5.3.   PERCENT BODY FAT FOR MEN

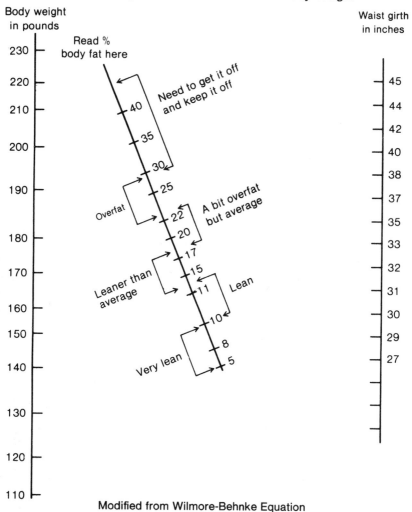

Percent Body Fat from Waist Girth and Body Weight

Modified from Wilmore-Behnke Equation

TABLE 5.4.   ANSWERS OF 2470 MEN TO "WHAT IS YOUR IDEAL WEIGHT?"

Height	Thin	Normal	Over-Fat
5′ 0″	113	116	146
5′ 2″	120	125	156
5′ 4″	127	133	166
5′ 6″	137	140	177
5′ 8″	145	150	188
5′ 10″	152	157	199
6′ 0″	160	166	210
6′ 2″	167	175	220
6′ 4″	175	184	230
6′ 6″	184	193	240
6′ 8″	193	202	250

"OH, MY ACHING FAT"

Eighty percent of the population—200 million Americans—have excess body fat. We know that about 70 million Americans are on diets each year, and we know for sure the diets don't produce thinness; they only cause more fatness. As the *Executive Fitness Newsletter* so aptly put it, "America has been on a diet for 25 years and has gained 5 pounds."

A good example of this occurred about two years ago. A 265-pound man came into our laboratory seeking advice on how to lose weight. After we explained the program to him, he decided not to participate because he didn't have the time to exercise. He spent his time on "fad diets." During the preceding year and a half, he had lost 30 pounds on the Stillman diet, 40 pounds on the drinking man's diet, and 60 pounds on the Scarsdale diet. That's 160 pounds and, according to my mathematics, he should have weighed about 100 pounds, but that's not how it works. We weighed him and he weighed 272 pounds. After all that misery, all that expense and all that ill health, he had not lost an ounce; in fact, he had gained 7 pounds in that one year.

Currently he is on an exercise program and on our stable nutrition plan. He weighs 218 pounds and is on his way down to about 165 pounds. There is no secret to the plan; he simply is controlling his diet and jumping on his rebounding equipment about 45 to 60 minutes, six days a week.

In our program at the university, we have had many similar success stories with men and women of all ages. Come join us in the next few chapters and find out exactly how you can lose those unwanted pounds of fat. And have fun doing it!

6

How Fit Is Your Body?

Fitness is not inherited. It requires regular vigorous exercise in order to be a reality. If you are like most Americans, you probably overestimate your level of cardiovascular fitness. From Figure 6.1 you can see that your level of activity, your age and gender determine just how fit you are. Scores achieved by vigorous exercisers are considered desirable.

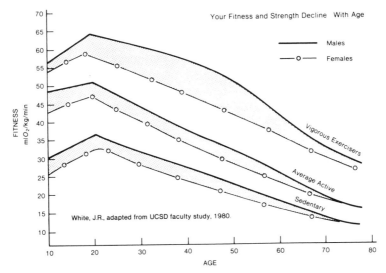

Figure 6.1. Cardiovascular Fitness.

The best measurement of fitness we have is the volume of oxygen your body can use when you're exercising at your maximum. The fitness number is expressed as VO_2 max (pronounced "VEE OH

TWO MAX"), with milliliters (ml) as the volume measurement. The results are divided by body weight so that large people don't get better scores just because they use more oxygen to do everything. The results are expressed in "milliliters per kilogram (of body weight) per minute"—ml/kg/min or $ml\,kg^{-1}min^{-1}$. In our lab we have measured fitness using a treadmill, a stationary bicycle and various rebounding equipment.

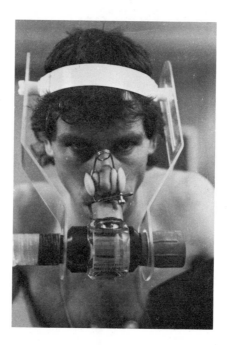

When you increase your VO_2 max, it represents an increase in the heart's ability to eject blood with each beat and an increase in the amount of oxygen consumed in the working muscles. Unfortunately, our VO_2 max decreases with age.

We are at our fitness peak at age 20 to 25. After that, it's all downhill. But wait! A quick look at Figure 6.1 shows that if you exercise regularly during the coming years, you will always be ahead of the average.

Figure 6.2 shows VO_2 max measurements for two individuals at different ages. One of the individuals got into our jumping program at age 50, while the other continued on a sedentary life. As you can see, after one year the exerciser improved his fitness level to a point greater than he had experienced at age 25.

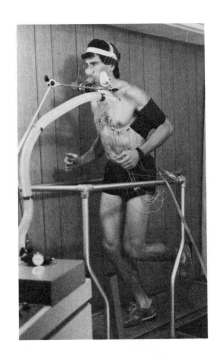

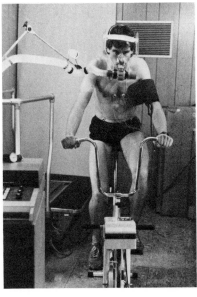

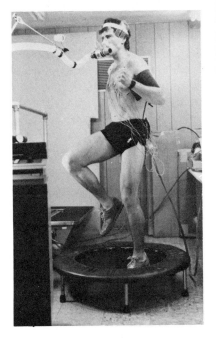

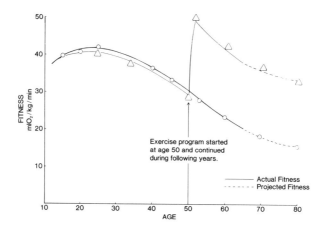

FITNESS
mlO₂ / kg / min

Exercise program started
at age 50 and continued
during following years.

——— Actual Fitness
------ Projected Fitness

AGE

Figure 6.2. Fitness Levels According to Exercise Habits.

REGULAR EXERCISE PRODUCES
IMPROVED FITNESS

Endurance exercises such as running, swimming, bicycling or jumping on rebounding equipment will produce an increase in your body's ability to utilize oxygen.*

The average sedentary American scores between 20 and 30 ml/kg/min. Look at Figure 6.1 again. If you wonder what your VO_2 max fitness score is and how you rate, read on!

How much you improve depends on your willingness to jump on a *regular* basis, how high the intensity of work, the duration of each session, sticking to it for a long time and the frequency of your exercise sessions. This program is designed to increase your fitness from 25–30 ml/kg/min up to 35–40 ml/kg/min after three to four months, and could increase it from 35 up to 45 ml/kg/min or more following six to nine months of training.

---

*We know that exercise will produce beneficial effects, but we also realize that overexercising is potentially harmful. So that you do not overexercise, we feel that a medical evaluation performed by a doctor, preferably one who is currently exercising himself, should be scheduled. The American College of Sports Medicine published advice for beginning exercisers over the age of 35 years. They state that regardless of your present health status, it is advisable to have a medical evaluation prior to a major increase in your exercise habits.

Now that you know what "VO$_2$ max" means, you'll probably want to know what your fitness number is. To go through the actual test, you would have to find a hospital or clinic that does the procedure. While being tested, you would run on a treadmill while breathing into a gas-analyzing machine. Additionally, you would have blood pressure readings recorded and heart rate tracings taken from instruments attached to the chest. It takes all day and can cost $200 to $850.

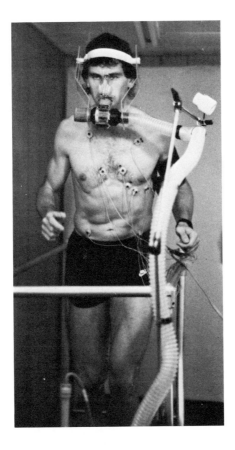

If you want to save the time and money, however, you can use the check-off fitness rating that we've developed. To use the check-off method, go to Tables 6.1–6.3, pages 54–56, and circle the number in each of the four categories that most accurately describes your present exercise practices. The tables are designed so that the sum of the scores in the four categories represents an excellent estimate of your VO$_2$ max.

TABLE 6.1. CHECK-OFF FITNESS RATING

To estimate your present fitness level, circle the appropriate number.

Age

	POINTS	
Your present age:	Men	Women
15–25	10	10
26–35	9	9
36–40	8	8
41–45	7	7
46–50	6	6
51–55	5	5
56–60	4	4
61–65	3	3
66–70	2	2
Over 70	1	1

Duration

The duration of your exercise sessions is:		
60 or more min.	18	14
50 min.	16	13
40 min.	14	12
30 min.	12	10
20 min.	10	8
10 min.	8	7
Less than 10 min.	5	5

Frequency

	POINTS	
How often do you exercise?	Men	Women
6–7 days per week	16	14
4–5 days per week	14	12
2–3 days per week	10	8
1 day per week	7	6
2–3 days per month	5	5
Infrequently or almost never	3	3

Intensity

The intensity or vigor of a typical exercise session is best described as:		
Sustained forceful breathing (160 heart rate, distance training)	24	21
Sustained vigorous breathing (150 heart rate, running at 7:30 mile pace, jumping vigorously)	21	17
Sustained brisk breathing (140 heart rate, running at 8–8:30 mile pace, jumping vigorously)	17	13
Intermittent forceful breathing (racquetball, squash, basketball, singles tennis)	15	14
Sustained comfortable breathing (130 heart rate, jogging, bicycling, swimming, jumping for joy)	15	14
Intermittent vigorous breathing (volleyball, softball, etc.)	14	11
Sustained light breathing (walking, hiking, jumping lightly)	11	8
Occasional very light exercise (golf, doubles tennis, gardening, etc)	9	6
No exercise	6	5

TABLE 6.2.   SCORING

ENTER YOUR SCORES HERE

Age   _____
Frequency   _____
Duration   _____
Intensity   _____
Total   _____ mlO$_2$/kg/min

This represents your estimated fitness level. If you are curious, see Table 6.3 to see how you rank with other people your age and sex.

TABLE 6.3   FITNESS RANKING

| | | FITNESS mlO$_2$/kg/min | | HEALTH PROFILE |
EXERCISE LEVEL	AGE	Men	Women	POINTS*
World Class	18–28	78–94	67–73+	18–19
[Very Highly Trained]	18–28	65–77	58–66	16–17
	18–25	62	53	
Highly Trained	26–35	60	51	
	36–55	58	49	12–15
[High Fitness Category]	56–69	52	44	
	70–79+	42	36	
	18–25	50	43	
Moderately Trained	26–35	45	37	8–9
	36–55	40	34	
[Average Fitness Category]	56–69	35	31	6–7
	70–79+	30	29	
	18–25	42	37	
Untrained	26–35	35	32	4–5
	36–55	30	28	
[Low Fitness Category]	56–69	25	24	2–3
	70–79+	20	19	

*See Health Profile on page 32.

Oh, yes, one more thought about VO$_2$ max, and for this, let's go back to Figure 6.1. We're going to use the case of a 40-year-old woman as an example, but the point can be made for any adult.

First, look at the VO$_2$ max that a sedentary 40-year-old woman can expect: about 24 ml/kg/min. Furthermore, it's never been lower in her life, and she's on the long slide. Now look what happens if she adopts a more active life-style, which puts her in the "average active" category. Her VO$_2$ max significantly increases to around 34 ml/kg/min, a higher value than she had when she was a sedentary 20-year-old. Even better, if she becomes a vigorous exerciser by vigorously jogging, swimming, aerobic dancing or jumping, her VO$_2$ max can increase to over 45 ml/kg/min. She'll feel younger than she has for many years—and she'll look it, too. Exercise like jumping for joy is the closest thing to the Fountain of Youth that we have!

7

Before We Jump—
Equipment and
Priorities

By this time, you know I believe jumping is a valuable exercise. It's fun and it will produce a fit, trim body regardless of age, gender or level of physical fitness, and it doesn't require much in the way of balancing skill beyond the average. The exercise is extremely valuable for folks who have not been active during the past, since it gradually allows you to increase your conditioning over a period of several weeks. In the next two chapters you'll learn how to adjust your exercise intensity by monitoring your heart rate. Then we'll introduce you to the exercise program, step by step, so you'll be able to begin in your own home. But before we go into the program, let's take some time to discuss clothing and equipment.

WHAT TO WEAR

If you choose to wear clothes while jumping, they should be loose and appropriate for the temperature. Most men need to wear shorts and a supporter. Women should wear shorts and a blouse. It is advisable for most women to wear a jogging bra, worn snugly but not so tight as to restrict free movement or shut off circulation.

Rubberized Suits

Despite the claims of their advertisers, wearing plastic clothing, rubberized suits or Saran Wrap while exercising or at rest is not recommended. While it is true that there's a temperature increase and more sweating, producing a reduction in total body weight (in the form of water loss), the reduction is temporary and dangerous because rubberized or wraparound material will cause the internal temperature of the body to rise beyond safe levels. Your body cannot cool itself in the normal manner and you may cook like a turkey. Your chances of dehydration and heat exhaustion are increased, and you may suffer an excessive washout of vital body minerals such as potassium.

Jumping should induce moderate to heavy sweating, which should be allowed to evaporate in the normal manner. It's easily absorbed into light cottonlike material found in T-shirts or blouses.

Shoes

Shoes are not essential unless the mat is slippery, and if shoes are worn, you should be fitted with a good pair of tennis shoes. Jogging shoes may not be sturdy enough. Wear soft cotton or wool socks, and if you are prone to blisters, rub a little Vaseline onto the "hot spots" on the foot before slipping on the sock.

THE BEST PLACE TO EXERCISE

Jumping can be performed anywhere, but I recommend that a spot be cleared of furniture or other objects for about 6 feet around each side of the rebounding equipment. It's advisable for beginners or those who have balancing problems to purchase a hand rail or secure some type of stabilizing hand grip or chairback (see page 8).

Jumping can be done indoors or outdoors and is probably done better on a carpeted floor or on grass. You should not place your equipment on slick or slippery surfaces as it has a tendency to slide. You may need to put a piece of carpeting or nonskid material under the legs of the equipment.

Jumping is especially fun when accompanied to fast music, so you might want to place your equipment near the stereo, radio or TV set. And by the way, it's always better to exercise to music with a friend. Many of our users say that they like to dance with a partner using a separate jumper device.

Care to guess what the latest craze is here in California? In some dance studios and YWCAs, women are joining afternoon "jumping classes," and while they bounce to a muted beat, they watch sexy soap operas. If you like the soaps, why not?

THE BEST TIME OF DAY
TO EXERCISE

You must select a time that can be set aside exclusively for exercise. From the point of view of safety, it is probably best not to exercise for at least two to three hours after eating a large meal. The best times would be in the morning before breakfast, just before the noon meal, just before dinner or two hours after eating dinner.

Many enjoy an early-morning exercise period before work, because they can rise, quickly dress, jump for a half hour, then shower and eat a leisurely breakfast. Others claim that exercising after work produces an increased vigor and alertness that improves their evening activities.

IS THERE A CORRECT WAY
TO JUMP?

The answer is that there is no specifically correct way to jump. Just remember to start slowly, gain balancing experience and don't fall off. As for the technique, many people use the jogging method, while others go for dance routines. Regardless of your choice, you will soon be able to jump to various types of music and be able to orchestrate imaginative and enjoyable exercise routines.

MUSCULAR FATIGUE AND JOINT
SORENESS

There are ways to reduce muscular fatigue and joint soreness and they are described below.

1. When jumping, keep your back comfortably straight, maintain good posture and "press the top of the head toward the sky." It's best not to constantly look at your feet, but gauge where you are on the mat by the sensations from your feet.
2. Your arms should be used for balance and held lightly at your side in an outward or upward position. Additional calories will be burned off if you use the arms to accentuate the movements of the entire body. Relax the upper arms and shoulders to avoid tightness.

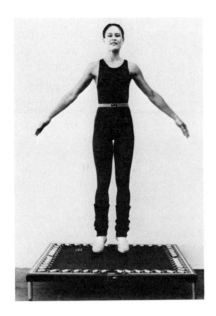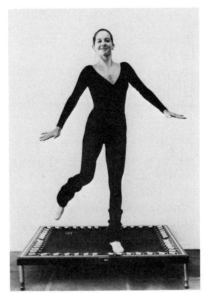

3. Breathe simultaneously through the mouth and nose.
4. The most common procedure is for the heel and the ball of the foot to strike simultaneously, and as you rebound from the mat, the toes are the last to leave the mat. You may also attempt to land on the balls of the feet, but this is not a natural way and is advisable only for the advanced jumper who wants to strengthen the front of the thigh muscles. This method may create soreness in the upper thighs.
5. If, while exercising, you become unusually tired, uncomfortable, confused, disoriented or experience unusual chest or arm pain, you should slowly stop your exercise and, if warranted, seek responsible medical attention.

THE BEST WAY TO START
THE PROGRAM

In the beginning, it is best to jump three to four days per week and follow your exercise heart rate as described in Chapter 8. You may be tempted to overexercise seven days a week and for up to 30 to 60 minutes per session. Don't overdo it; in fact, in the beginning you might want to alternate days of exercise with days of rest to decrease fatigue and lessen the possibility of injury.

After several weeks of exercise, the bones, ligaments and muscles of the legs, ankles and feet will be adequately conditioned to support your body weight, so that daily extended periods of jumping can be scheduled. On the days that you do not jump, we recommend that you do some stretching or calisthenics, and some alternate forms of exercise such as swimming, stationary bicycling, walking or slow jogging. Your total program includes five basic parts, which will be explained fully in Chapter 9.

REBOUNDING EQUIPMENT

Each year the American public is served up a new fad diet or new fad exercise device. These fads pass into obscurity only to be rediscovered and renamed three to five years later. Rebounding equipment, however, is more than a fad. The reason is that it is so simply designed that it is gimmick-proof. You still have to do the exercise, but the rebound equipment can make it more fun and less traumatic to jump.

There are several jumping devices on the market, either in sports equipment shops, through mail order or direct-selling distributors. I have found that no single device deserves a special endorsement or condemnation. You can shop with an eye for suiting your own needs and pocketbook. However, be wary of cheap imitations. They are poorly constructed, break easily and deliver an inferior bounce.

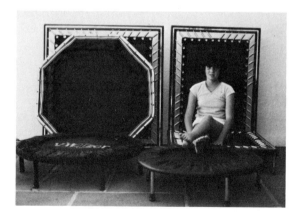

Size varies from 30 to 48 inches in diameter, and both square and round designs perform equally well. The legs, which are threaded, welded or bolted on, support the frame 8 to 10 inches from the floor, and the devices are sturdy and stable enough not to collapse or tip under normal use. Most units we have tested in the laboratory have been subjected to extensive and rigorous work representing 20–30 years of normal home use.

The spring for the jump is supplied by either coil springs or a heavy rubber shock cord, and the mats are usually made of an almost indestructible synthetic cloth. We've had people weighing over 250 pounds using the jumping devices in our laboratory on a regular basis with no mishaps.

When you shop for your own jumping gear, the best advice is to take off your shoes and try it out. However, if you've never been on one before, be a little careful in the showroom and remember that these devices aren't designed for acrobatics, so they will seem very "stiff" to a novice.

"MENTAL SET"—A FINAL THOUGHT ON PRIORITIES

A sedentary person who decides to put exercise into his or her life is making a major life-style change. When we look back on the progress of the people in our jumping classes after six months, we see that most of them have succeeded and are exercising joyfully, that some have failed and are back to their sedentary habits, and some feel coerced but are still exercising while resenting every minute of it.

What's the difference? Well, at the beginning they all wanted to be in the "joyful" group—at least they said they did. Why did some make it into a joyful activity and some not?

The best answer is that the winners started with a better "mental set." By mental set, we mean that the new exercisers who were successful prepared themselves before they started by examining their reasons for beginning exercise, setting priorities and goals and arranging their attitudes and exercise schedules so that it was a reward, not a punishment.

So, before we go any further, let's look at some goals, some priorities and some of the sources of fun and support that you can arrange to make jumping a joy.

We all know that exercise is good for us, but it's also true that during a busy day exercise is often the activity given up. The following list may be helpful in getting you into the exercise program and keeping you there.

Make a check beside each question to which your answer is "yes."

1. Do you want to:
   Lose weight? ____
   Strengthen your muscles? ____
   Become physically fit? ____
   Protect yourself against heart disease? ____
   Just have fun with exercise? ____

2. Are you willing to dedicate a little time, on a daily basis, to improve the areas checked above? ____
   Do you believe exercise really helps? ____
   Are you willing to put in the necessary time? ____
   To lose weight, will you exercise regularly and eat properly? ____

3. It's helpful to discuss these issues with someone you trust, to actually make a verbal commitment to stick to the program for at least four weeks. And try to complete three to six months of exercise.

4. Don't fall prey to the "I'll start tomorrow" syndrome. Remember, every day you follow the program you will lose one-sixth of a pound of fat.

5. Keep your rebounding apparatus near the TV or the stereo so that every time you pass it, you can take a few extra jumps.

6. Contact groups of people or individuals or friends who are exercisers and try to form friendships.

7. Be patient with yourself. It took five, ten, perhaps twenty years or more to get out of shape. So take six months to a year to get back into shape. Don't give up because of an occasional setback.

8. If you miss a day or more, simply get back on the program as soon as is reasonably possible. If you do have a minor setback, don't feel guilty. Don't get depressed and sit around getting fat, remorsing over the fact that you haven't exercised. That's simply adding injury to injury and fat to fat. Reduce your stress, guilt, and anxiety by exercising the next available opportunity and continue from there. You *can* do it!

9. On those days when you don't feel perfect, you may want to start your slow warm-up exercise, and if, after completing five minutes, you still don't feel good, call it quits for the day. There is always another time.

On those times when you don't especially feel like exercising, consider these options: (1) If you are truly ill and feel that you may have a medical problem, it is best not to exercise—rest and see your physician; (2) if you just don't feel like exercising due to a lack of interest or motivation, think back to the goals and benefits that you set for yourself, and remember that the roll of fat around your middle will most likely shrink a bit if you exercise, and will probably swell a bit if you just call it quits for the day.

After you have been into the exercise program for several months, you will probably become an evangelist yourself. You'll be tempted to preach, lecture your friends and cite the virtues of exercise. However, the best plan would be simply to ask them if they wish to exercise and refer them to this book as a way to start their program.

If you feel you're ready to go for your program, read on. Chapters 8 and 9 will put you into action!

8

Your Exercise Heart Rate—A Perfect Speedometer

Your exercise intensity is determined by how vigorously you perform during your jumping session. To be safe, your intensity should be determined by your age and your present fitness level. You must choose an intensity great enough to improve fitness and reduce body fat, but not so vigorous as to be dangerous.

Your body has a great speedometer to let you know whether you are exercising at an appropriate intensity—your heart—and this is achieved by monitoring the heart rate during exercise. You can easily determine your heart rate by locating the radial artery, pressing lightly on the wrist about one-half inch above the thumb and counting the number of beats for six seconds. Multiply the count by ten to get the heart rate per minute.

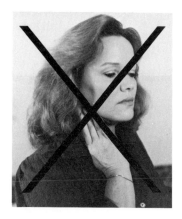
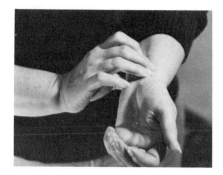

When counting your heartbeats, remember to watch your time-piece for a full six seconds. As the sweep second hand passes the starting point, you must count the first pulse you feel as "zero," the next pulse as "one," the next as "two," and so on. Continue counting for the full six seconds. The "zero" pulse starts the interval for counting. Practice a few six-second counts before reading on. (See Figure 8.1.)

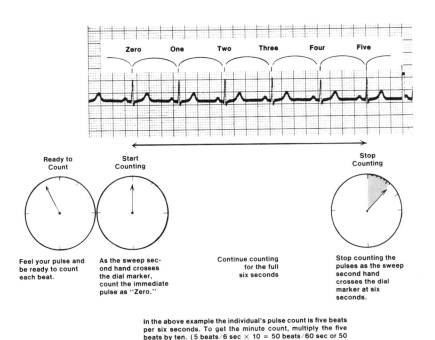

Figure 8.1. Six-Second Pulse Count.

As you begin to exercise, even at low levels of intensity, your heart rate should immediately begin to rise. After several minutes of slow warm-up exercise, your heart rate will tend to plateau and will remain at that steady state as long as you don't increase your exercise intensity. As you increase your intensity, your heart rate should also increase. It is natural and quite expected that each time you increase the work level, the heart rate would increase in a like manner.

If you are not in good shape, your heart rate may increase rapidly during the first minute or two of exercise, and it is then advisable to stop, take a quick six-second count and make sure that you have not exceeded your prescribed exercise heart rate. After several weeks of regular exercise, you will probably notice that you have to work a little harder in order to achieve the heart rate that was so easily achieved weeks before. This is good—it means you're getting in shape!

As you might guess, after you've been exercising for a month or so, you will be able to work at fairly high work loads for extended periods of time with a relatively low heart rate. Why? Because your heart, lungs, blood vessels and muscles are more efficient, resulting in greater productivity for less work energy.

THE BEST HEART RATE DURING EXERCISE

It is difficult to give you an exact exercise heart rate without seeing you in person. However, Tables 8.1 and 8.2 show the exercise heart-rate range within which you should keep your heart rate during exercise.

For example, if you are a 40-year-old female without heart disease, a little overweight, and have had a fairly sedentary life, using the check-off fitness ratings from Chapter 6, you will probably rank in the low-fitness category. To determine your exercise heart rate, simply locate your age on the chart, slide your finger to the right until you come under the column marked "Low Fitness," and you see that your exercise heart rate is between 14 and 15 beats per six-second count. This corresponds to a heart rate of between 140 and 150 beats per minute. (Remember that you're going to be keeping track of your heart rate through six-second counts, and all the numbers on the chart are for six seconds.)

After you have been in the program for about three months, you might refer back to Chapter 6 and repeat the check-off fitness rating. If you then score up in the average-fitness category, you might wish to select an exercise heart rate for your age and gender from the "Average Fitness" heart rate column. For the 40-year-old female looking under "Average Fitness," the new exercise heart rate would be between 140 and 160 beats per minute, or 14 to 16 beats for a six-second count.

Since you are different from any other person, you may find that, although the check-off rating places you in the average-fitness category, jumping at that exercise heart rate might make you out of breath and uncomfortable. Should this occur, adjust yourself over to

TABLE 8.1. EXERCISE, WARM-UP, AND COOL-DOWN HEART RATES FOR WOMEN (RECORDED FOR 6-SECOND PERIOD) *

Age	Exercise Heart Rate	Warm-up Cool-down Heart Rate
Low Fitness		
12–24	16–17	12–13
25–38	15–16	11–12
39–52	13–14	10–12
53–66	12–14	9–10
67–72	11–13	8–9
over 72	10–12	7–8
Average Fitness		
12–24	16–18	13–14
25–38	15–17	12–13
39–50	14–16	11–12
51–63	13–15	10–12
64–75	12–14	9–10
over 75	11–13	8–9
High Fitness		
12–18	16–19	
19–22	16–19	13–14
23–28	16–18	13–14
29–33	15–18	12–14
34–42	15–17	12–13
43–50	14–15	11–13
51–60	13–15	11–12
61–69	13–14	10–12
70–75	12–13	9–10
over 75	11–13	8–10

*Multiply the heart rates by 10 to find minute rates (e.g., 13 × 10 = 130 beats per minute).

a lower fitness category, and select a more comfortable exercise heart rate according to your age and gender. The chart is simply a guideline; your exercise heart rate should always be based upon the way you feel when you jump. When you are exercising, you should be able to carry on a conversation without gasping or running out of

TABLE 8.2 EXERCISE, WARM-UP, AND COOL-DOWN HEART RATES FOR MEN (RECORDED FOR 6-SECOND PERIOD)*

Age	Exercise Heart Rate	Warm-up Cool-down Heart Rate
Low Fitness		
12–19	15–16	12–13
20–32	14–15	11–12
33–46	13–14	10–12
47–60	12–13	9–10
61–72	11–12	8–9
over 72	10–11	7–8
Average Fitness		
12–20	16–17	13–14
21–34	15–16	12–13
35–46	14–15	11–12
47–58	13–14	10–12
59–69	12–13	9–10
over 69	11–12	8–9
High Fitness		
12–18	17–18	13–14
19–30	15–16	12–14
31–42	15–17	12–13
43–52	14–16	11–12
53–66	13–14	10–12
67–72	12–13	9–10
over 72	11–12	8–9

*Multiply the heart rates by 10 to find minute rate (e.g., 13 × 10 = 130 beats per minute).

breath. It is also important that you stop periodically during your exercise session and take a quick six-second heart rate count to determine if you are over or under your exercise heart rate. If you are not on your exercise heart rate, adjust your pace accordingly.

Also, there is a tendency to jump happily along at a comfortable pace that is too low a level for full benefit. This is usually well below your exercise heart rate, so take a quick six-second count and increase your pace and intensity if necessary.

9

The Exercise Program

This chapter contains a great deal of material, but don't be intimidated. Read the chapter once all the way through, and then return to Figure 9.1 below, and the schematic drawing on page 96. You'll see that the whole five-phase exercise program can be easily understood in terms of that drawing. You might want to cut out or reproduce that page and pin it up where you keep your clothes or equipment.

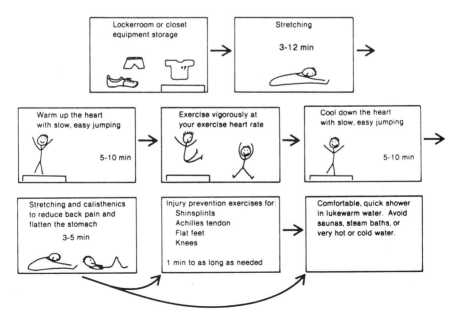

Figure 9.1. The Whole Program—A Quick Look.

First of all, let's describe the *five* basic elements of each exercise session. To become fit and limber quickly, to avoid injury and to get the most out of the program, each of these five elements should be incorporated into every exercise session.

1. *Stretching and joint motion*   Employing slow full-range movements of the major muscles and joints.
2. *Warming up the heart*   Mild warm-up exercise designed to enlarge the arteries of the heart and prepare the muscles of the body for more vigorous exercise.
3. *Exercising the heart*   Jumping on your rebounding equipment at your exercise heart rate for a specific length of time.
4. *Cool down the heart*   Mild exercise designed to bring the heart, blood pressure and muscle activity into a gentle recovery state.
5. *Calisthenics*   To restretch the muscles that have gotten stronger and shorter during jumping, to strengthen and flatten the stomach muscles and to stretch specific muscles to prevent low back pain.

STRETCHING AND JOINT MOTION

The following stretching exercises are designed to safely and comfortably prepare you for the more vigorous exercise to follow. The stretches start at the feet and work up to the neck. Table 9.1 contains the specific stretch routine, the body position and the number of minutes needed to complete each of the 13 stretches.

During the first several sessions, you'll have an easy time if you sit on your rebounder or on the floor, open the book to the stretching exercises and follow the instructions word for word. Allow for a little extra time until you learn the routine. (By the way, should any stretch be uncomfortable, don't feel obliged to keep it in your routine.)

Let's get on the rebounder and try each stretch; later you'll be able to zip through them in less than ten minutes.

TABLE 9.1. STRETCHING AND JOINT RANGE OF MOTION*

| | | MINUTES REQUIRED | | |
EXERCISE	BODY POSITION	*Beg.*	*Int.*	*Adv.*
A. Ankle and foot flexibility	sitting	1 min	1 min	1 min
B. Ankle circles	sitting	$\frac{1}{2}$ min	$\frac{1}{2}$ min	1 min
C. Ankle extension	sitting	$\frac{1}{2}$ min	$\frac{1}{2}$ min	$\frac{1}{2}$ min
D. Straight ankle pull	sitting	$\frac{1}{2}$ min	$\frac{1}{2}$ min	$\frac{1}{2}$ min
E. Buttock stretch	lying on side on floor	10 reps	15 reps	20 reps
F. Side leg lifts	lying on side on floor	15 reps	25 reps	30–40 reps
G. Trunk flexion	sitting	1 min	$1\frac{1}{2}$ min	2 min
H. Mad cat	crawling position	1 min	1 min	1 min
I. Lazy jog in place	standing	$\frac{1}{2}$ min	$\frac{1}{2}$ min	$\frac{1}{2}$ min
J. Side stretcher	standing	$\frac{1}{2}$ min	$\frac{1}{2}$ min	$\frac{1}{2}$ min
K. Ladder climb	standing	$\frac{1}{2}$ min	$\frac{1}{2}$ min	$\frac{1}{2}$ min
L. Arm circles	standing	1 min	1 min	1 min
M. Neck rotation	standing	$\frac{1}{2}$ min	$\frac{1}{2}$ min	$\frac{1}{2}$ min
	TOTAL TIME	9 min	10 min	12 min

*All stretching exercises should be executed slowly (in a nonballistic manner) and should utilize full range of joint motion.

STRETCHING EXERCISES

A. Ankle and foot flexibility (rotation, flexion and extension)

1. Sitting position, one leg straight, other leg crossed over top of thigh.
2. Grasp toes with one hand.
3. Rotate fully in both directions, flex and extend for 15 seconds.
4. Switch legs and repeat routine for 60 seconds.

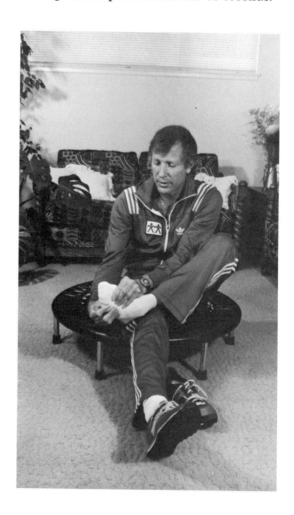

B. Ankle circles

1. Sitting position, legs straight, heels touching floor.
2. Simultaneously rotate ankles in clockwise direction for 15 seconds.
3. Rotate ankles in counterclockwise direction for 10 seconds.
4. Continue rotating ankles for 30–60 seconds.

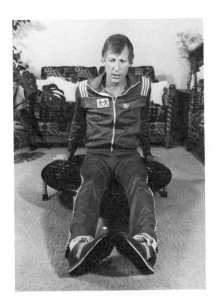

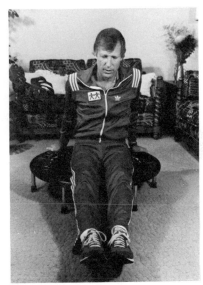

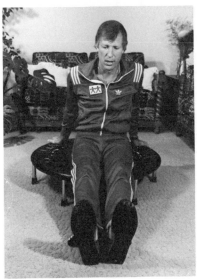

C. Ankle extension/flexion

1. Sitting position, legs straight, heels touching floor.
2. Fully extend ankles, point and curl toes and hold for 5 seconds. Flex toes up and hold for 5 seconds.
3. Repeat extension and flexion but this time point toes outwardly; hold for 5 seconds.
4. Repeat extension and flexion but this time point toes inwardly; hold for 5 seconds.
5. Continue for 30–60 seconds.

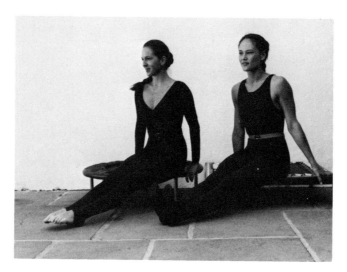

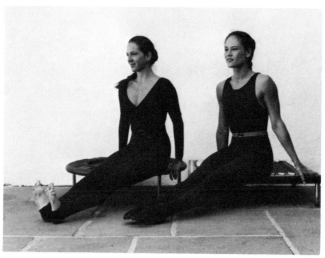

D. Straight ankle pull

1. Sitting position, knees bent, heels on floor, grasp toes.
2. Slowly straighten one leg until fully straight, pull back on toes, hold for 5 seconds.
3. Return leg to bent position and simultaneously straighten opposite leg; hold for 5 seconds.
4. Repeat 5 times.

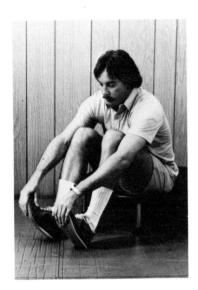
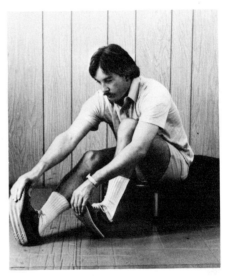
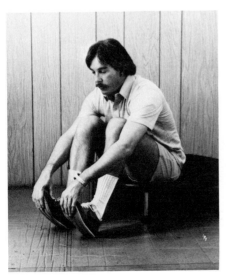
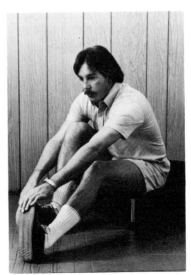

E. Buttock/thigh stretch

1. Lying on side.
2. Grasp top knee with top hand and raise knee toward chest.
3. After touching knee (thigh) to chest, relax leg and slide hand down to ankle and pull ankle to rear, stretching front of upper leg.
4. Repeat ten times and then turn to opposite side and repeat.

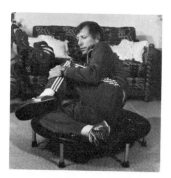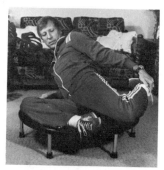

F. Side leg lifts

1. Lying on side, holding legs straight, toes pointed.
2. Lift top leg maximally, keep straight, hold for 2 seconds.
3. Return to resting position and repeat 20 times.
4. Turn to opposite side and repeat routine.

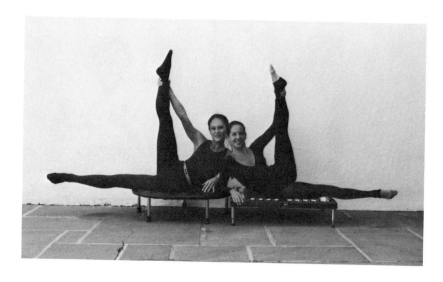

G. Trunk flexion

1. Sitting position, feet together, legs straight, hands holding rear thighs near ankles.
2. Bend forward slowly, grasping the back of the knees, and slowly attempt to put face to knees; exhale as you come forward.
3. Hold for 5 seconds.
4. Repeat 12 or more times.

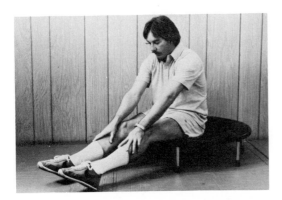

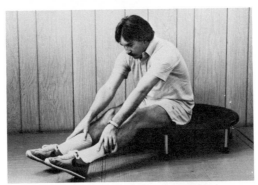

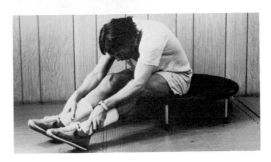

H. Mad cat

  1. Crawling position, hands, knees and toes on floor.
  2. Stretch by arching spine as high as possible; exhale.
  3. Hold for 5 seconds and relax to starting position.
  4. Repeat 12 or more times.

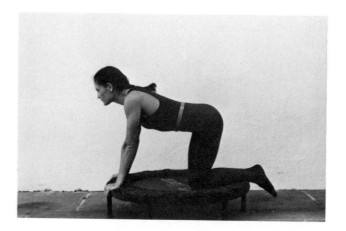

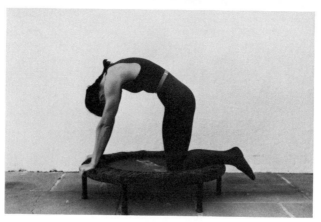

I. Lazy jog in place (shake-out)

1. Standing position, hands at side and relaxed.
2. Slowly jog in place at a rate of 74 steps per minute.
3. Deep relaxed breathing and, if you wish, slow rotation of head.
4. Continue for 30–60 seconds.

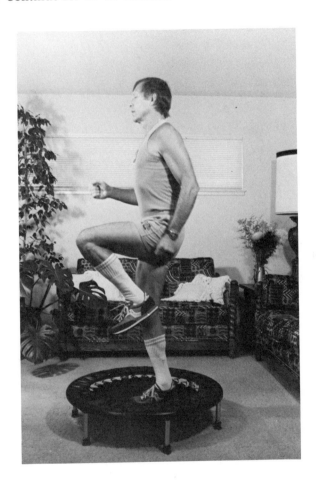

J. Side stretcher

1. Standing or kneeling position, arms extended above head.
2. Grasp right wrist with left hand, pull and bend slowly to left; hold for 5 seconds.
3. Return to starting position and grasp opposite hand and bend to the opposite side; hold for 5 seconds.
4. Repeat 6–12 times.

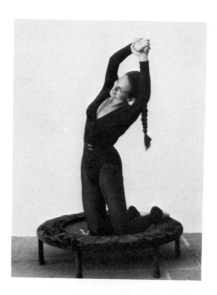

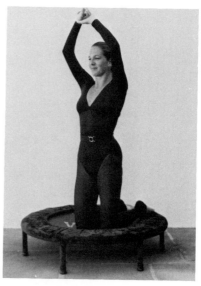

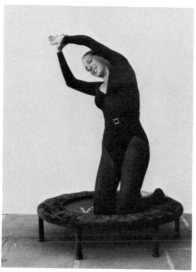

K. Total body stretcher (ladder climb)

1. Standing position, hands above head.
2. Raise up on toes and alternately pull down with one hand at a time, simulating a ladder climb.
3. Repeat for 30–60 seconds.

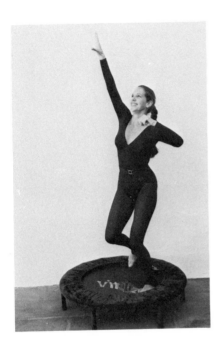

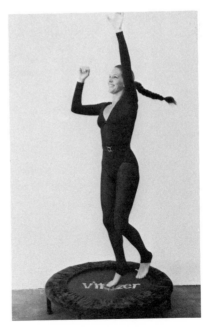

L. Arm circles

1. Standing or kneeling position, arms at side.
2. Slowly rotate and stretch arms as in the backstroke for 10 seconds.
3. Next, rotate arms as in the front crawl for 10 seconds.
4. Repeat for 40–60 seconds.

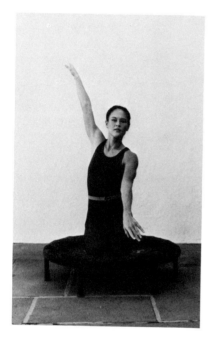

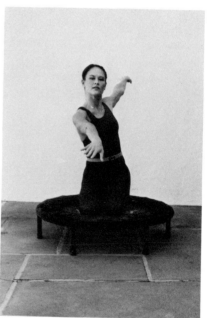

M. Neck rotation

1. Position of attention.
2. Rotate neck with either the chin, ear or back of head in near-contact to the chest, shoulder or back.
3. Rotate in opposite direction.
4. Continue rotation for 30–60 seconds.

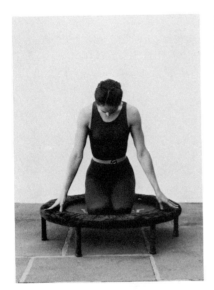
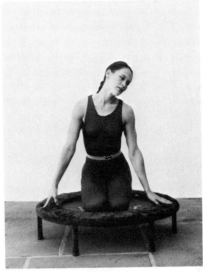
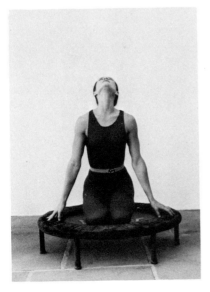
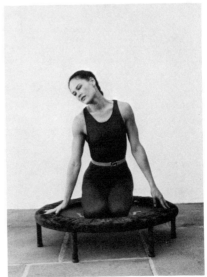

WARMING UP THE HEART

Now that you've finished your stretching, step up on your rebounding equipment, get a comfortable stance and we'll guide you through jumping a simple bounce and then some jogging.

1. Stand with your feet as wide as your shoulders. Relax your shoulders and let the arms swing freely as you start a gentle bouncing motion.
2. Keep your toes in contact with the mat and allow your heels to bounce a couple of inches off the surface. This is called the bounce.

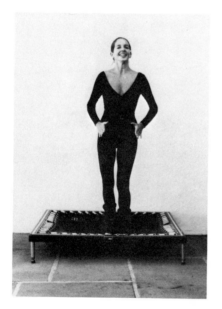

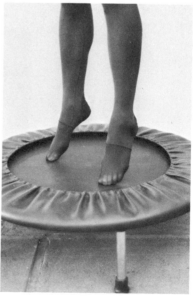

3. Continue this simple bounce until you feel comfortable. Next, while keeping the toes in contact with the mat, alternate bouncing from one foot to the other. This is called jogging or marching.

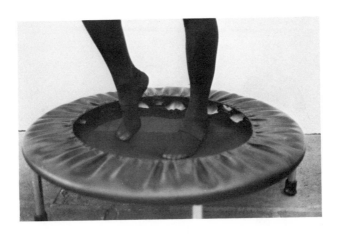

4. Now switch back to the simple bounce and, if you feel comfortable, increase the vigor by bouncing deeper into the mat and allowing the heels to leave the mat while keeping the toes in contact with the surface. With more experience you will soon be able to bring your feet completely off the mat.

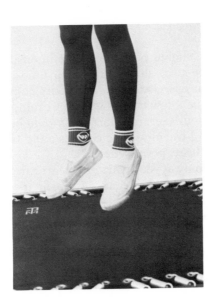

5. When you feel comfortable with this, switch back to the jogging and allow the alternating feet to leave the mat an inch or two. With a bit more experience, you will be able to bring the feet completely off the mat and comfortably raise up the knees.

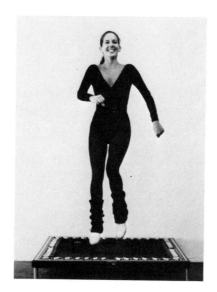
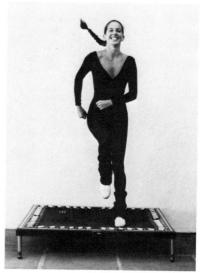

Your jumping should be of moderate intensity and continuous. After a minute or two, stop and take a quick six-second count. Remembering your exercise heart rate from Chapter 8, the warm-up heart rate should be a few counts less. For example, if you are a 40-year-old woman, your exercise heart rate would be 14 to 15 beats per six seconds. During warm-up, the count should be one to two beats lower, or 11 to 12 beats per six seconds.

Continue jumping at your warm-up heart rate for five to ten minutes. Warm-up is important because it opens the arteries that feed blood to your heart. It should be vigorous enough to increase the heart rate well above the resting heart rate, but not so vigorous as to reach your exercise heart rate.

During your five- to ten-minute warm-up, take at least two different six-second heart rate readings to make sure you are at your warm-up heart rate.

EXERCISING AT YOUR EXERCISE HEART RATE

During the first few weeks of jumping, you will start with just a few minutes of exercise, and progressively increase the length of time you jump over the weeks. If you find that your heart rate is above the exercise heart rate, continue to exercise but reduce the intensity a bit. After a few days of jumping you will be able to maintain your exact exercise heart rate almost unconsciously.

During the first few weeks, the length of time that you maintain your exercise heart rate will be small, and each subsequent week thereafter the duration will increase about a minute or so. Take a quick look at Tables 9.2 and 9.3 so that you will understand how you progressively increase the amount of exercise time.

TABLE 9.2.   EXERCISE PROGRAM FOR MEN— DURATION OF EACH EXERCISE SESSION IN MINUTES

Week	Exercise Heart Rate (Beats per six seconds)					
	10–12	*13*	*14*	*15*	*16*	*17*
1	3	5	8	8	8	10
2	4	6	9	9	9	12
3	5	7	10	10	10	14
4*	6	8	12	12	12	16
5	7	9	14	14	15	18
6	8	10	15	16	17	20
7	9	11	16	18	19	23
8*	10	12	17	20	21	25
9	11	13	18	22	23	28
10	12	14	19	23	25	30
11	13	15	20	25	27	32
12*	14	16	21	26	29	34
13	15	17	22	27	31	36
14	16	18	23	28	33	38
15	17	20	24	29	34	39
16*	18	20	25	30	35	40

*Reevaluate your fitness level and determine a new, higher exercise heart rate if needed (pages 54–56; 68–70).

TABLE 9.3. EXERCISE PROGRAM FOR WOMEN— DURATION OF EACH EXERCISE SESSION IN MINUTES

Week	Exercise Heart Rate (Beats per six seconds)						
	10–12	13	14–15	16	17	18	19
1	6	10	16	16	16	16	16
2	7	12	18	18	18	18	18
3	8	14	20	20	20	20	21
4*	10	16	24	24	24	24	25
5	13	18	27	27	27	27	28
6	15	20	30	30	30	30	31
7	17	22	32	33	33	33	34
8*	19	24	34	35	36	36	39
9	21	26	36	37	39	39	42
10	23	28	38	39	41	41	45
11	25	30	40	41	43	44	48
12*	28	32	42	43	46	47	50
13	30	34	44	45	49	50	53
14	32	36	46	48	51	53	57
15	34	38	48	50	53	56	60
16*	36	40	50	52	57	60+	60+

*Reevaluate your fitness level and determine a new, higher exercise heart rate if needed (pages 54–56; 68–70).

Let's go back to our example of a 40-year-old woman for a moment. Her exercise heart rate is 14 to 15 beats per six seconds. Following her five-minute warm-up at a heart rate of 11 to 12 beats per six seconds, she will then maintain her exercise heart rate for 16 minutes each session, and during the second week she will increase that up to 18 minutes of exercise each session. For week number three, it will be 20 minutes of exercise, etc.

The frequency of exercise should be five to six days per week, keeping in mind that the more one exercises, the more effective the program. It is best not to miss two days in succession, as the benefits of the prior workouts will be partially lost.

Enter your warm-up heart rate, your exercise heart rate and your cool-down heart rate below (see pages 68–70 if you don't recall your heart rates).

Five to ten minutes of warm-up at a
heart rate of: _____beats / six seconds

Exercise at a heart rate of: _____beats / six seconds

Five to ten minutes of cool-down at
a heart rate of: _____beats / six seconds

After completing your scheduled number of minutes of jumping at your exercise heart rate, you should not stop exercising abruptly. Instead, reduce the intensity and relax the body so that your cool-down heart rate will be about the same as your warm-up heart rate. If you stop jumping too abruptly, blood pooling might occur and cause mild shock, hyperventilation, and muscle cramps.

STRETCHING AFTER YOU JUMP

Often after you finish aerobic exercise, the rear thigh muscles and lower back muscles actually shorten in length. This may lead to an abnormal pelvic tilt, resulting in low back pain. To prevent this type of low back pain, the following three stretches have been effective in our laboratory:

N. Trunk flexion

1. Sitting, feet together, legs straight, hands at side.
2. Bend forward, grasping the knees or ankles, and slowly press forward.
3. Hold for 5 seconds.
4. Return to original position.
5. Repeat for 1–2 minutes.

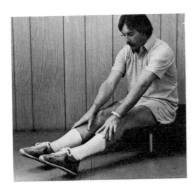
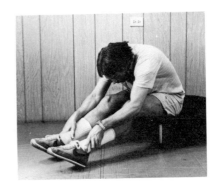

O. Straight leg pull

1. Sitting position, knees bent, heels on floor, grasping toes.
2. Slowly straighten one leg until fully straight, pull back on toes, hold 5 seconds.
3. Return leg to bent position and simultaneously straighten opposite leg; hold for 5 seconds.
4. Repeat for 1–2 minutes.

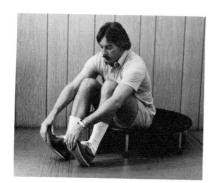
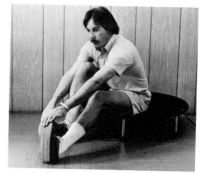
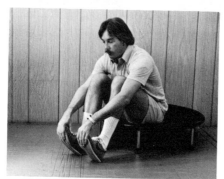
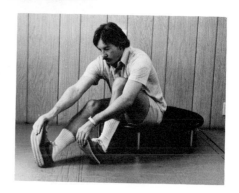

P. Bent knee sit-up

1. Lie flat on back, knees bent approximately 45° and wide apart, hands folded on chest.
2. Bend at waist, bring left elbow forward and place on opposite knee. Slowly return to floor.
3. Bend at waist, bring both elbows as far forward as possible. Slowly return to floor.
4. Bend at waist, bring right elbow forward and place on opposite knee. Slowly return to floor.
5. Repeat 10 to 20 times for beginners, 21 to 35 times for intermediates and 36 or more for advanced exercisers. Some advanced exercisers complete more than 200 each day.

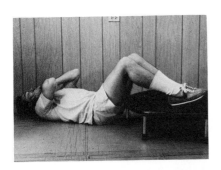
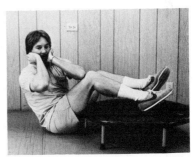
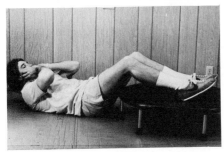
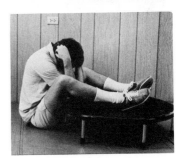
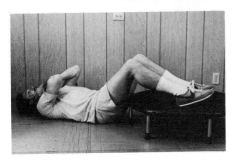
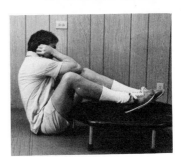

ENERGY EXPENDITURE

So far, we promised that jumping will help control your weight. Well, it's true—using jumping as exercise burns calories, but you're probably wondering how many.

For each exercise session the number of calories burned will depend upon how many minutes and how vigorously you jump. For example, looking at Figure 9.2, you can see that when you exercise at a heart rate of 135 beats per minute (13 to 14 per six-second count), you will be burning calories at a rate of between six and ten per minute. If you are a small person, weighing around 120 pounds, you will be burning about six calories per minute. If you weigh 180 pounds, you will burn about ten calories per minute.

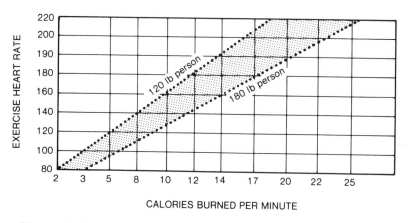

Figure 9.2. Approximate Caloric Burn-off During Jumping for Joy at a Given Heart Rate.

To determine *total* calories burned during your exercise session, simply multiply the time in minutes that you maintain your exercise heart rate by the number of calories per minute. For example, if you jump at a heart rate of 135 for 20 minutes, and you weigh around 180 pounds, you would simply multiply ten calories per minute by the 20 minutes, which would be a total of 200 calories for that session. In short, if you hold your exercise heart rate steady, 8 to 10 minutes of jumping equals 1 mile of jogging, 16 to 20 minutes of jumping is worth 2 miles of jogging and 24 to 30 minutes of jumping represents the same caloric expenditure as running 3 miles. In other words, every ten minutes of jumping or every mile of running equals 100 calories.

If you exercise five to six days per week, that moderate amount of exercise would allow you to lose nearly 18 pounds of body fat during the next year. If you combined that with the nutrition program outlined in Chapter 12, you could lose approximately 40 pounds in 12 months.

You may be tempted to increase the duration of your sessions because you'd like to lose fat more rapidly. It has been our experience that by following the outline in this chapter, you will be able to maintain your interest, avoid premature fatigue, and not become stiff and sore. It took you a few years to get out of shape and over-fat, so why not take a comfortable 12 weeks to get yourself back into reasonably good shape.

A usual question asked, "Could I do two exercise sessions a day?" The answer is yes, if you follow the week-by-week exercise program and leave adequate time for rest between sessions, you will not overextend yourself and will double the caloric burn-off and double your pleasure as well.

Figure 9.3 shows heart-rate changes and caloric burn-off before, during and following your jumping exercise. Notice that during rest the heart rate is about seven beats per six-second count (70 beats/minute). About one calorie per minute is burned off at rest.

1. *Stretching and range of motion*   Heart rate varies between eight and ten beats per six seconds and the caloric burn-off is 2 to 3 calories per minute.
2. *Warming up the heart*   Comparable to brisk walking, the heart rate increases to 11 to 12 beats per six seconds. The caloric burn-off is 3 to 4 calories per minute.
3. *Exercising*   Here the heart rate increases to 13 to 14 beats per six seconds and the caloric burn-off is 6 to 10 calories per minute.
4. *Cooling down the heart*   Heart rate comes down to about 11 beats per six seconds and the caloric burn-off is 5 to 6 calories per minute.
5. *Postexercise stretching and calisthenics*   Heart rates vary between 9 and 12 beats per six seconds. The caloric burn-off is 2 to 3 calories per minute.

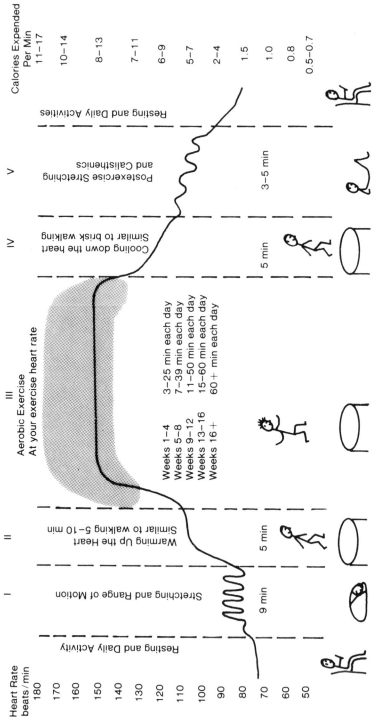

Figure 9.3. Heart Rate and Caloric Changes During 5-Point Exercise Session.

MAKING JUMPING FUN

Before we get into additional jumping techniques and routines, I want you to know one of the reasons that I jump nearly every day is that I can watch the news on television or listen to fairly loud, upbeat music. I have purchased a moderately priced stereo to go with my jumping gear and even use a stereo headset. With your jumping, use music, music, and more music! It'll keep you coming back for more.

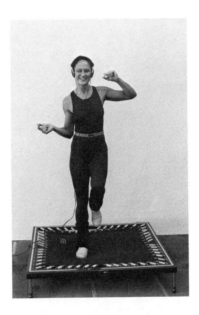

When jumping, keep your body erect and keep your shoulders level but relaxed. The arms and hands may be used for balance, but the movement should be smooth, gentle and not too jerky. Breathing should be deep and comfortable and, as you inhale and exhale, breathe through the nose and the mouth simultaneously. The entire body should feel light, and the energy should be focused during each rhythmical bounce. Each rebound should provide a joyous lift, and the foot contact should be solid and unwavering. Your arm movements should be flowing and energetic and add to the rhythmical flow of the movement.

During the simple bounce (feet striking the mat simultaneously) the number of foot contacts should be between 90 and 132 per minute:

90 bounces per minute is minimal (burns 2–4 cals/min)

100 bounces per minute is moderate exercise (burns 3–5 cals/min)

110 to 115 bounces is brisk exercise (burns 4–8 cals/min)

120 bounces per minute is vigorous exercise (burns 6–10 cals/min)

132 bounces per minute is exhaustive exercise (burns 9–14 cals/min)

During jogging (single footsteps), the range is between 100 and 200 steps per minute:

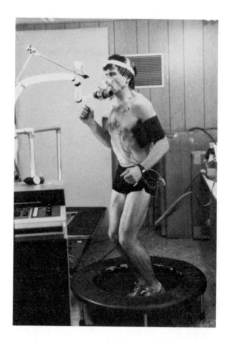

105 steps per minute is minimal exercise (burns 2–3 cals/min)
115 steps per minute is moderate exercise (burns 2–4 cals/min)
125 steps per minute is moderately brisk (burns 3–4 cals/min)
140 steps per minute is very brisk (burns 4–8 cals/min)
150 steps per minute is vigorous (burns 6–10 cals/min)
180 steps per minute is very vigorous (burns 9–13 cals/min)
200 steps per minute is exhaustive (burns 10–15 cals/min)

Jumping for joy includes all varieties of aerobic rebounding maneuvers: jumping, bouncing, jogging, marching (usually performed to military music), twisting, "jumping jacks," double jogging or double bouncing, pointing, kicking, slapping, ladder climbing, skipping rope, aerobic dance, ballet, jazz dance and skiing.

Jumping activities can be done singly or combined into multiple movements. For example, you might bounce five times, followed by slow jogging, followed by five bounces, followed by four kicks, followed by ten seconds of twisting, etc. The following photos and sketches should assist you in developing routines that are fun and safe.

LET'S BE CREATIVE

Ballet

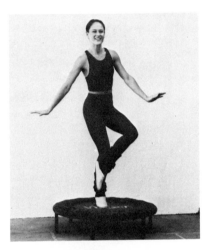

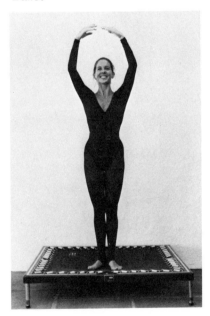

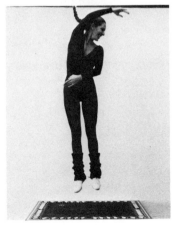

Rope Skipping

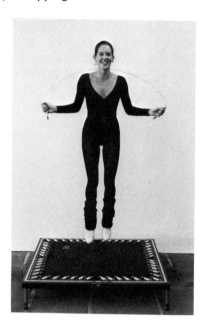

Rope Skipping for the Advanced

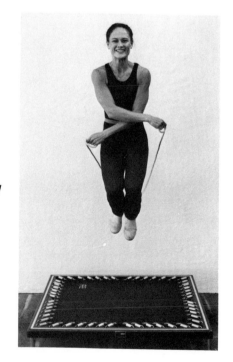

Disco Boogie

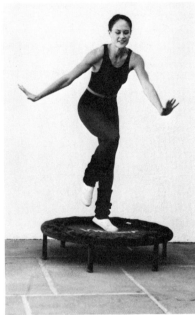

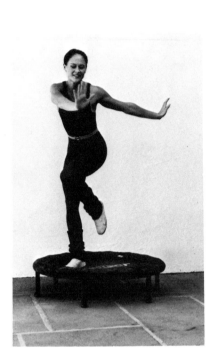

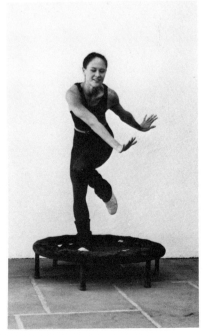

All That Jazz

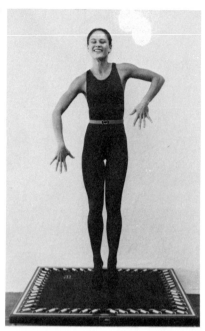

Modern Dance

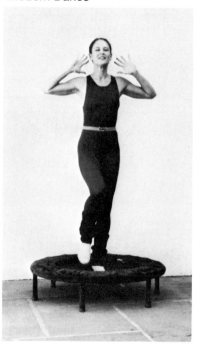 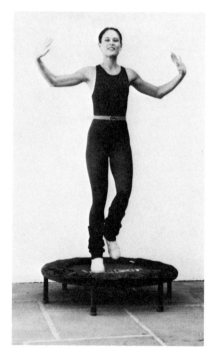

Aerobic Dance

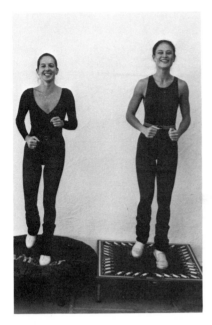

Foot Slap

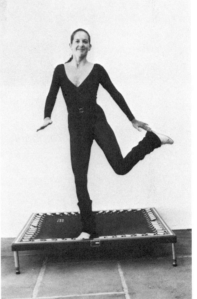

Twist

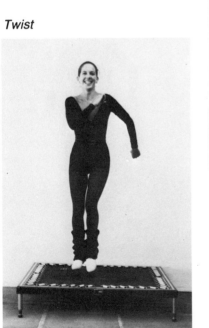

Towel

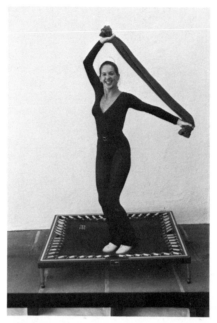

Tamborine

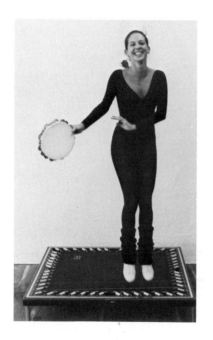

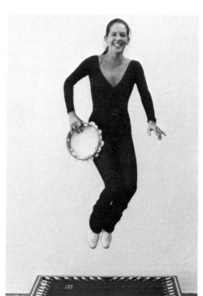

Fanny Bounce

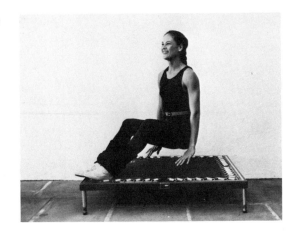

Jump-N-Jacks

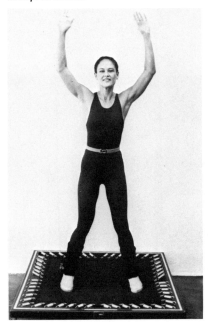

Judo Chops

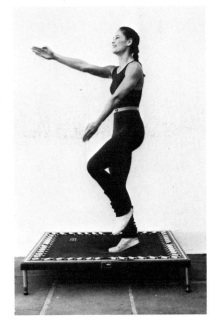

DANCE MOVEMENTS

Basic Bounce

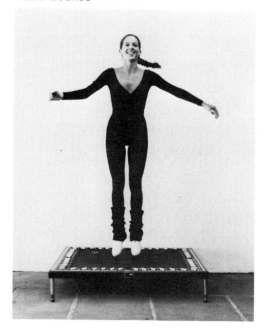

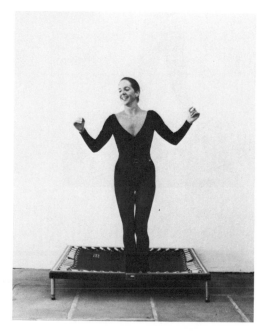

Side Kick, Bounce, Side Kick. . . .

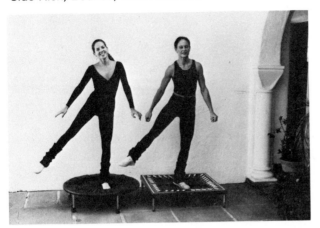

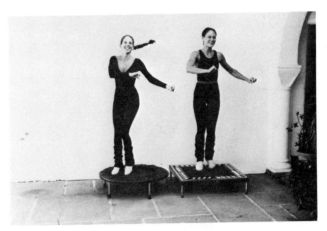

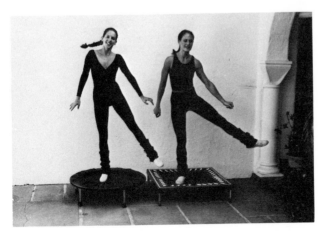

Low Twist

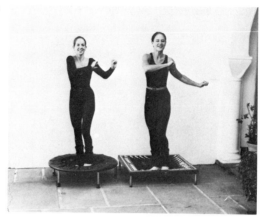

High Twist

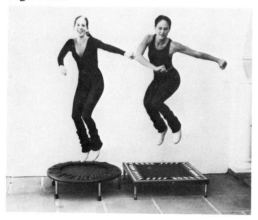

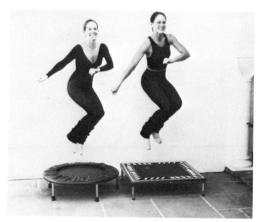

Bounce (hands high), Bounce (hands low). . . .

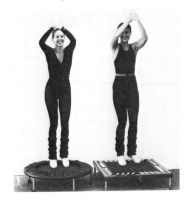
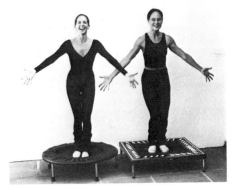

Front Kick (hands low), Bounce (hands high). . . .

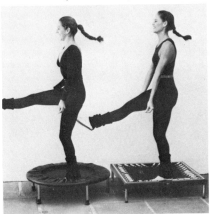
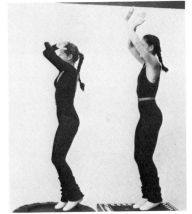

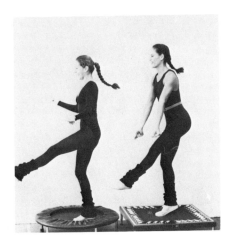
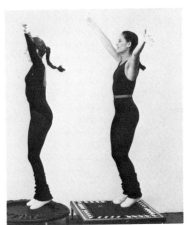

Bounce (arms right), Bounce (arms high), Bounce (arms left). . . .

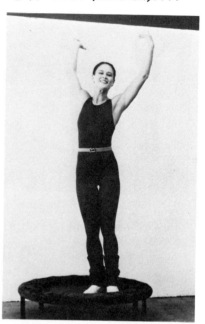

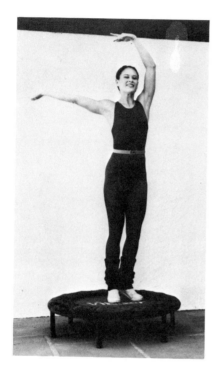

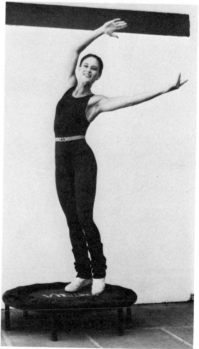

DANCE ROUTINES

Linking Your Dance Movements into a Continuous
Aerobic Dance Routine

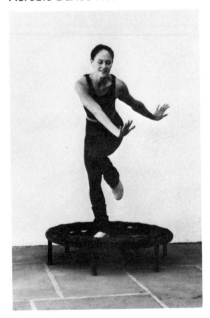
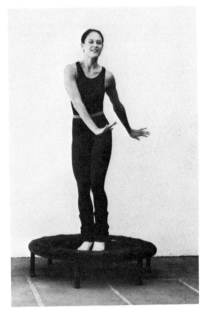
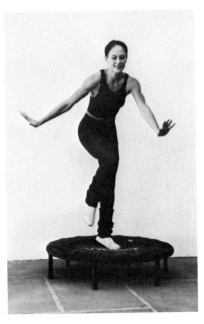
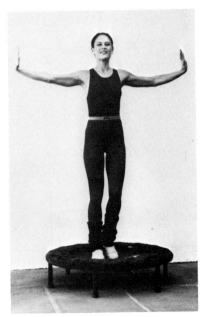

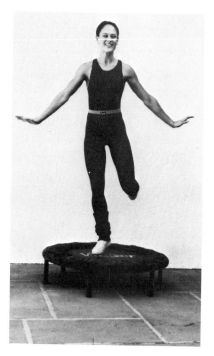
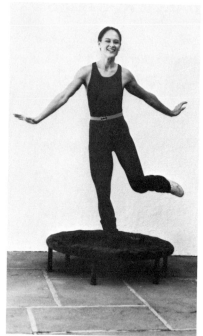
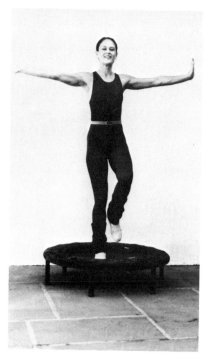
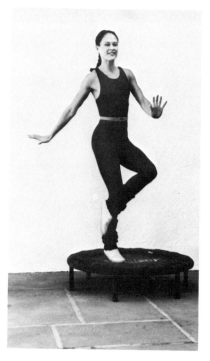

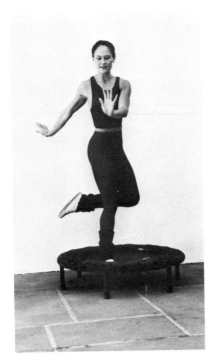

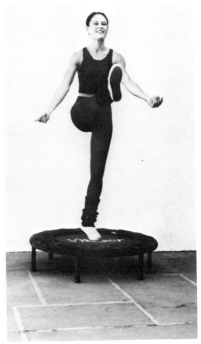

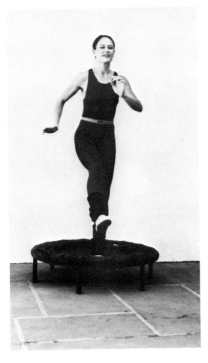

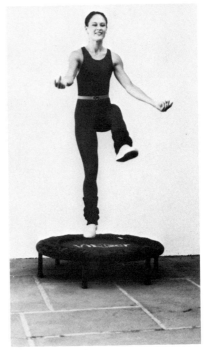

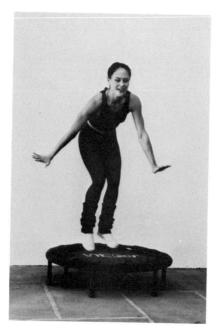

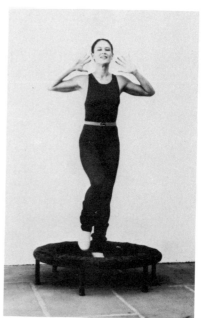

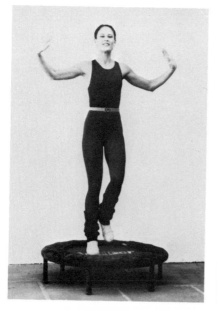

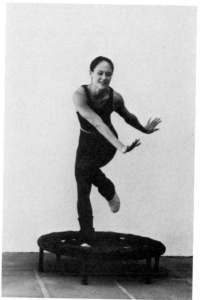

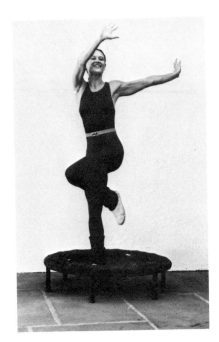
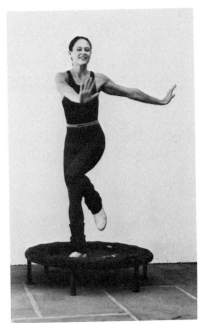
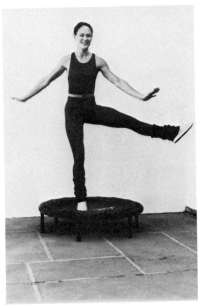
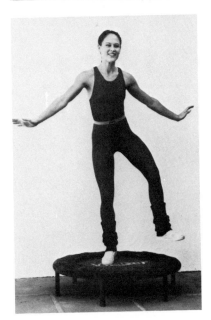

Finish with a Smile!

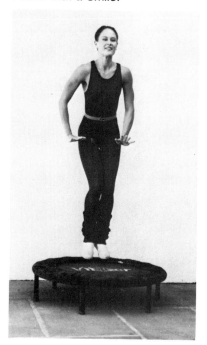 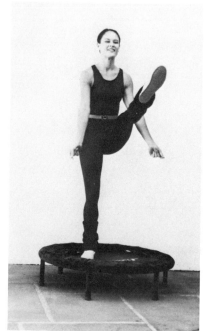

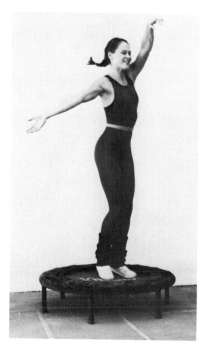 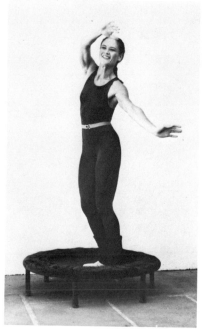

IMPROVE YOUR SPORTS AND BALANCE

Home Run Fever

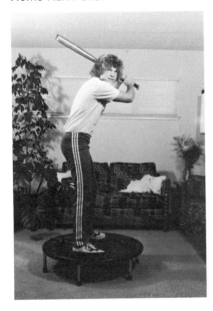

"Tennis Anyone?"

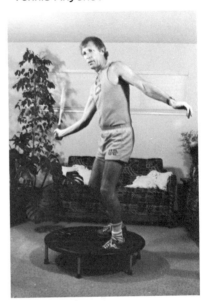

Boxing and Other Martial Arts

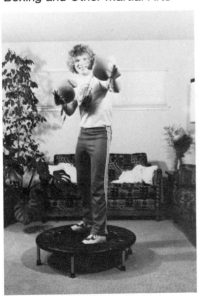

Racquetball

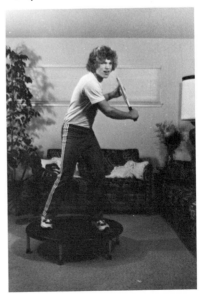

"En Guarde"

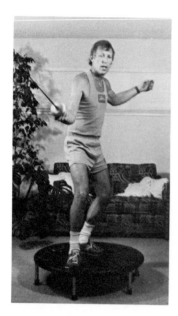

"Touché"

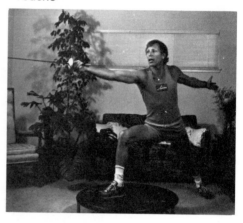

Jumping with Weights

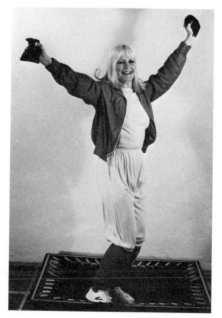

FUN AT ALL AGES

Warm-up

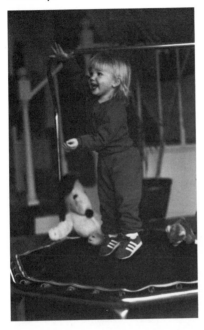

Exercise

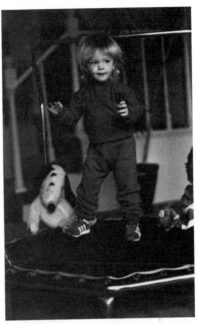

Cool-down

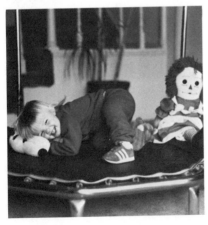

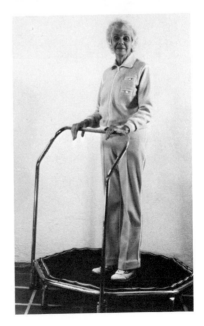

BUSINESS EXECUTIVES AND CHILDREN

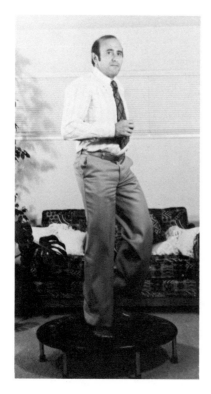

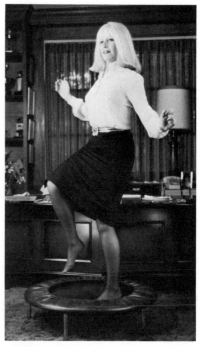

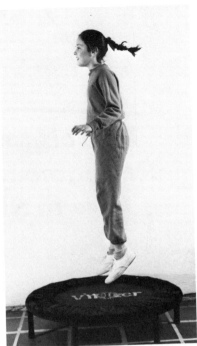

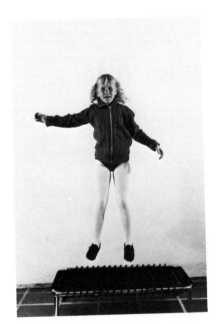

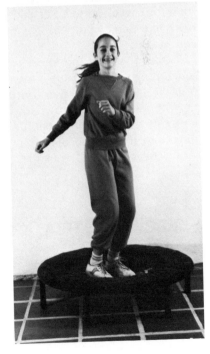

10

Exercise Hints, Tips, Recommendations, and How to Stay with It

Many jumpers have said that jumping is the most relaxing and enjoyable exercise they have ever tried, and since it's such fun and so healthy, it would be good to stay with it. The best way to stay with it is to set some short-range goals and maintain your exercise program for a four-week period. Set aside the time on your schedule, however busy, and don't let anything come between you and your rebounding equipment.

Once that first four-week segment is over, you will discover that scheduling time for your jumping is worth the while. After the first four weeks, go for another four-week segment. This will get you over the "initial jump," and by then you will have developed some behavior skills that will allow you to continue your program through the third and fourth and fifth four-week segments, until it becomes an indispensable part of your life.

EXERCISE MOTIVATION

During the first four-week segment, you will probably be adequately motivated. Toward the end of the second four-week segment, that enthusiasm may be waning and you may search for ways to get out of exercise. We're going to give you some clues on how not to defeat your good intentions by answering some commonly asked questions.

What should I do when something important takes the time I've set aside for exercise?

Go ahead and meet the emergency, but reschedule your exercise the next morning and again that evening to make up for the lost time. The best idea is to schedule your exercise at a time of minimal disruption.

What happens if I get sick?

While you're ill, don't exercise. As soon as you're feeling better, look at your exercise schedule and slip back a week or two so that you'll be exercising fewer minutes than you were at the time you became ill. The main thing is to start again after your illness.

What if I'm injured?

If it's serious, see your physician. If you can safely determine that a physician is not needed, then rest for an adequate number of days and back up a week or two on your exercise schedule.

What if I'm out of town?

Well, I do have friends who routinely carry their rebounding equipment with them on trips when they go by air. I know of dozens who travel by car and would not think of going on a business trip or vacation without their rebounding equipment.

In fact, several have stated that when they're driving along the freeway and become bored, tired or sleepy, they pull over to a rest area, drag out their rebounding equipment, turn up the car radio and bounce for 10 to 15 minutes. Then, feeling wide awake, they continue driving for another hour or so.

How do I avoid the feeling that I'd just as soon put off exercise until tomorrow?

The reason you feel this way is that you probably have other things on your mind that seem pressing. Remember, both your body and mind need diversion and activity. So jump to music and you will probably not be bored and not want to put it off until tomorrow.

However, if this should occur, we have designed the following exercise schedule that proceeds week by week and day by day. Jot down the number of minutes you jump each day and total the number of minutes at the end of the week. Then compare that to the optimal number of minutes. If you try that for four weeks, I think your "do it tomorrow syndrome" will disappear.

EXERCISE SCHEDULE

Record the number of minutes of jumping for joy you completed at your exercise heart rate.

Week	Mon	Tues	Wed	Thurs	Fri	Sat	Sun	Total	OPTIMUM NUMBER OF MINUTES PER WEEK		
									Beg.	Int.	Adv.
1									25–35	35–45	50–100
2									25–35	40–50	55–110
3									30–35	45–55	60–120
4									30–40	50–60	65–125
5									35–45	55–65	70–130
6									40–50	60–70	73–135
7									45–55	65–75	80–140
8									50–60	70–80	85–145
9									55–65	75–85	90–150
10									60–70	80–90	95–155
11									65–75	85–95	100–160
12									70–80	90–100	105–165

Week	Mon	Tues	Wed	Thurs	Fri	Sat	Sun	Total	Beg.	Int.	Adv.
13									75–85	95–115	110–170
14									80–90	100–110	115–175
15									85–95	105–115	120–185
16									90–100	110–120	125–190
17									95–105	115–125	130–200
18									100–110	120–130	135–210
19									105–115	125–135	140–220
20									110–120	130–140	145–230
21									115–125	135–145	150–240
22									120–130	140–150	155–260
23									125–135	145–155	160–270
24									130–140	150–160	165–280
25									135–145	155–165	170–290
26									140–150	160–170	175–300
52									180–250	200–275	300–400

A Little More Help to Insure Success

Here is a list of things that have helped people achieve great success in jumping.

1. Follow the schedule listed on pages 124 and 125.
2. Make it a positive habit, and it will enliven your life-style.
3. Jump to music or to television.
4. Exercise with a friend or in a group.
5. Tell others of your new exercise program, particularly family, work associates and lovers.
6. Keep a record of your progress as described above.
7. Don't be afraid to reward yourself.

In fact, at the end of the first four-week segment, I want you to turn back to this page and reward yourself with some type of treat. So that you will know what the reward will be, I want you to list four rewards, gifts or treats that would be appropriate rewards for maintaining your health program.

1. _____ Weeks 1–4
2. _____ Weeks 5–8
3. _____ Weeks 9–12
4. _____ Weeks 13–16

BREATHING WHILE YOU EXERCISE

The more vigorously you exercise, the more rapidly and deeply you will breathe. You will find that the major energy expenditure is used when you are exhaling. As you increase your breathing, you will increase the number of breaths per minute and the amount of air coming in and going out of the lungs. At rest, you breathe about 12 times per minute. During brisk exercise that goes up to about 20 to 25 times per minute, and during maximal exercise you breathe 30 to 35 times per minute.

Air should be inhaled and exhaled through the nose and mouth simultaneously. Don't think about your breathing; simply breathe on demand and as frequently as you desire. While jumping on your rebounding equipment, you may be tempted to breathe in rhythm with your bounces. If this is comfortable, it's okay. Holding your breath during exercise is not recommended, nor is very rapid, quick breathing of any benefit. Slow and steady breathing is desired, and some researchers have stated that a slightly more forceful inhalation, followed by a longer and softer exhalation, is beneficial in order to relax. Try it and see what you think.

MUSCLES THAT GET SORE

If you follow the exercise program that we have designed for you, you probably will not encounter much muscle soreness or tightness. Occasionally, however, during early exercise sessions, the rear calf muscles may feel minor pain. If this should happen, slow your pace for a while, and over the coming days your muscles will condition themselves and the pain will subside.

Should you ever experience a muscle that is sore from spasm or have a muscle cramp, one of the best ways of relieving it is by stretching the muscle lightly but firmly for two to three minutes. Should you experience cramps in the rear calf muscles, simply sit down on your equipment and perform the straight ankle pulls for a minute or two (see page 77). This should relieve the cramp.

MORE QUESTIONS AND ANSWERS

Is sweating good?

Yes, sweating is good for you. In fact, if you're not perspiring, you're probably not exercising vigorously enough. However, you should be aware that sweating causes a loss of the natural electrolytes of the body. These electrolytes include sodium and potassium. Also, if you're taking diuretics for water loss, the water that is lost contains potassium, and excessive removal of potassium either from diuretics or sweating may cause a feeling of fatigue or uneasiness. A good way to restore potassium levels is to eat a few pieces of any fruit or two to three servings of fresh or frozen vegetables, grains, legumes and unsalted seeds and nuts.

How does jumping for joy help ex-athletes?

During the competitive season, it's not uncommon for male and female athletes to consume about double the number of calories that are consumed by nonathletes. An extra 500 to 2000 calories may be consumed by an athlete, but most of that is burned away during the strenuous training program each day. When the athlete's season or career comes to an end, the number of calories consumed tends to stay the same, but the caloric burn-off is greatly reduced. The energy (fat and sugar in the blood) that is not being used for exercise "looks around" for a place to be stored and is deposited in the ex-athlete's fat cells.

Ex-athletes must remember that a combination of daily exercise and a prudent diet is effective in maintaining optimal weight. If you're an ex-athlete, keep to a specific time to exercise each day, gradually reduce your calorie intake and be especially careful of fats and sweet foods in your diet.

Should I monitor my heart rate when I exercise?

It's probably best to monitor your heart rate. If you find that you have exceeded your exercise heart rate, continue the exercise but at a slower pace. Exercise is safer if you monitor your heart rate.

Are recreational sports good?

Almost any type of physical activity is good for you. Some are just better than others. For example, jogging, swimming, bicycling, aerobic dancing and jumping give the most benefits in terms of weight loss and protection against heart disease. However, there are other activities in life and those include golf, social dancing, bowling, sailing, horseback riding, gardening and many others. These activities should supplement, but not be a substitute for, your daily aerobic exercise activity of jumping. These activities are considered recreational because they do not promote adequate fitness. Some are good for burning off calories, if you are willing to play 18 holes of golf or an hour of tennis or walk for 60 minutes per day.

If you're interested in burning off calories in order to lose weight, there are other ways and they include walking upstairs instead of taking the elevator and parking several blocks from your job or office and then walking to work. Each week you might park your car a block or two farther away from work until you're walking 30 minutes to work and 30 minutes back to the car. Another method to reduce calories would be to take a walk prior to eating lunch or dinner, knowing that some exercise before eating may reduce your hunger.

This next idea may seem a little embarrassing, but when you take a friend out for dinner or lunch, you might order an extra salad and split the meal. I know of many very affluent people who routinely split a dinner with their partner. You will leave the restaurant satisfied but not stuffed. Most typical dinners eaten out will have calories found in two home-cooked meals. And, finally, pass up those interoffice party snacks of cookies, candy, doughnuts and other tidbits. You don't need them.

Short Hints and Recommendations for Jumping Exercise

1. *How often?* Minimum of four days a week, optimum of five to six days a week.
2. *How long?* Follow your schedule with an eventual goal of 20 to 40 or more minutes of continuous aerobic exercise.
3. *Equipment?* Shoes or no shoes: loose, comfortable fitting clothes. Avoid rubber suits, wraparounds and anything that does not allow the body to cool itself during exercise.
4. *Muscle soreness?* Should not occur, but if it does, continue working out on a slow progression on a daily basis. Stretching will reduce soreness and muscle spasm.
5. *Dizziness or chest pain?* In very rare cases, chest pain or dizziness may develop during exercise. Should this occur, the activity should be stopped and the person put to rest. A physician should be consulted before restarting the exercise program.
6. *Fatigue following exercise?* Fatigue lasting two hours or more following the end of exercise is an indication that the intensity or duration may have been too much. Jumping should leave you with a sense of pleasant relaxation and not fatigue. If you have perspired a lot, you might want to eat some fresh fruit to replace the potassium lost during heavy sweating.
7. *Faithful adherence?* The best idea is to exercise almost every day, and try not to miss two days in a row.
8. *Competition?* Don't try to compete with anyone except yourself. Follow the exercise plan in Chapter 9 and proceed slowly and wisely.

SMOKING

In Chapter 4 we said that we would talk about quitting smoking later. Well, now is "later." But before those of you who smoke start feeling threatened, remember your "mental set," calm down and read on. The methods offered for quitting are meant to help you. And like everything else recommended in this book, these methods have been tried successfully by thousands of people.

The effects of tobacco are so devastating and the extent of the damage it causes is so far-reaching and profound that it must be of major concern. The unfortunate thing is that the tobacco habit is so compelling that it will require a major effort on your part should you decide to quit. The methods of quitting are:

1. *Quitting "cold turkey"* is traumatic, difficult; will work for some and not for others.
2. *Cut the number* of cigarettes you are presently smoking in half each month. For example, if you are currently smoking 30 cigarettes per day, starting tomorrow and for the next 30 days permit yourself to smoke only 15 cigarettes per day. Count out 15 cigarettes in the morning, put them in your pack and smoke them at any time during the day, but that's the limit for the day. During the next month, cut the number down to eight cigarettes per day. Each morning dole out eight cigarettes in your package and, again, smoke them any time during the day that you choose, but remember that for that day you only smoke those eight.

   In the third month you cut the number down to four cigarettes per day, and in the fourth month, two cigarettes per day. At the end of that month you quit smoking totally.
3. *Cut the nicotine* in half by changing the brand you smoke. If you presently smoke a high-tar, high-nicotine cigarette, switch to a cigarette with only half the tar and nicotine for a month. During the second month, switch to one of the lowest-level tar and nicotine brands available. You will be tempted to smoke more cigarettes. Fight the urge; you want to reduce your level of addiction, so it will be easier to quit later.

Now let's look at some hints that will help you with the withdrawal symptoms. Since you have a nicotine addiction, all the cigarette does is to reduce the withdrawal feeling. If you put your cigarette consumption on a regular schedule, you may have to experience some of that withdrawal pain, but at least you know that at some time you will be able to satisfy that with a cigarette. A couple of rules that will be helpful follow.

1. Never smoke in your house. When you do smoke, go to the patio or garage and stand. Do not relax with television or a good book or a cup of coffee; we need to break the pleasure and reward states that have been associated with smoking.
2. Remove your cigarettes and your ashtrays from around the telephone. Many people automatically light up a cigarette when the phone rings.

3. Do not smoke while riding in a car. Smoke only in the standing position and away from other people.

There are a lot of reasons why you should stop smoking, but the best are always personal, and if you wish to think those over and write them down, it might be of help to you. Oh yes, for you women, the latest statistics show that women who smoke and drink coffee have a 60 times greater chance of developing breast cancer. Kind of a high price for a little smoke and brown water.

11

Preventing Injuries

There are two types of sports injuries. The first are traumatic body-contact injuries that occur in sports like football, boxing and ice hockey. The second type of injury is an exercise-related injury that occurs to runners, tennis players and any other athletes in sports where joints and muscles are repeatedly strained.

In our rehabilitation laboratory at UCSD we have found that exercising on rebounding equipment produces very few injuries. For example, in our study we found that joggers, basketball players, tennis players, racquetball players and other athletes who perform on hard surfaces are at high risk for injury. In activities such as walking, swimming, stationary bicycling, rowing and jumping, the injury rate is very low.

Injuries that occur to the feet, ankles, knees, legs and hips can be minimized by using low-weight-bearing exercises, such as jumping, because the impact against the foot is absorbed over a greater period of time. The impact experienced in mild jumping is no greater than that you would experience in walking on a level, carpeted floor.

Even though the impact is low, we would like to share with you some ideas on how to prevent injuries in your new jumping program:

1. *Always stretch before exercising.* The majority of injuries occur following inadequate stretching. The stretching technique discussed in Chapter 9 will help minimize injuries.
2. *Overuse.* This simply means that when you begin your exercise program, you could start off too fast or exercise too long at a time. It is best to follow your exercise plan.
3. *Early warnings.* Be aware and sensitive to small twinges of pain or bodily discomfort. The best advice is "listen to your body," and if it hurts, don't exercise. If the pain is persistent,

see a physician. And, most important, should you develop chest pain or similar symptoms when you're exercising, stop your exercise and consult a physician.

SPECIFIC INJURIES, REHABILITATION AND PREVENTION

Arch sprains or flat feet. These sprains are usually the result of constant stress or repeated pounding on pavement. For joggers they may result in a change in the types of running shoes or running surfaces, or a change in stride techniques. Arch sprains rarely occur from rebounding. If the injury occurs, the immediate treatment would be the application of ice compresses and elevation. After medical consultation, you may wish to start an arch exercise program. Treatment for arch sprains and strains is nearly identical to those exercises prescribed for flat feet. The following exercises have been successful in strengthening the muscles that support the foot and arch.

A. Marble pickup

1. Sitting position, barefoot, paper wads on floor (size of large marbles).
2. Pick up pieces of paper by forcefully gripping with toes, hold for 5 seconds, drop paper to floor.
3. Repeat with opposite foot.
4. Continue for 3–5 minutes

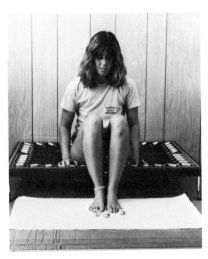
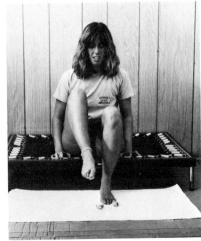

B. Towel pull

1. Sitting position, barefoot, towel on floor, a 2- to 5-pound weight on towel.
2. Grip towel with toes and alternately pull with toes completely past heels.
3. Continue for 3–5 minutes.

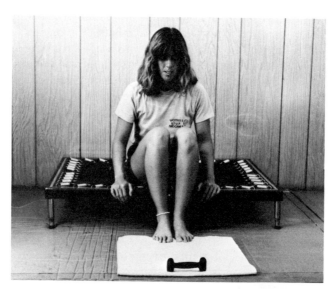

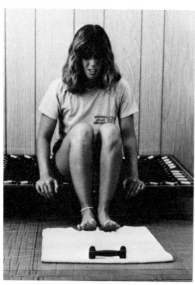
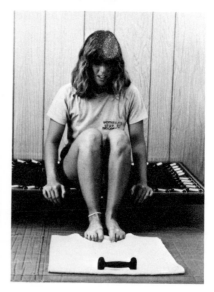

C. Towel push away

1. Sitting position, barefoot, a 2- to 5-pound weight on towel placed on floor behind heels.
2. Grip towel with toes and alternately move towel completely past toes and away from body.
3. Continue for 3–5 minutes.

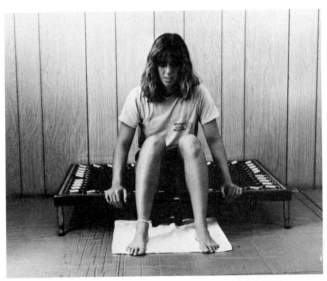

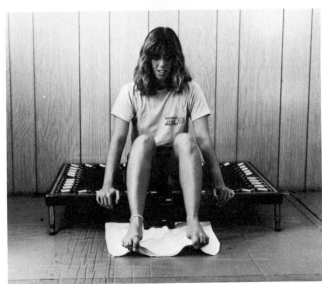

D. Achilles tendon stretch (pes planus—flat feet)

1. Standing 1 foot from wall, hands on wall.
2. Extend one leg back 3–4 feet with heel on floor, bend front knee.
3. Move trunk forward slowly to a point of bearable stretch retaining heel–floor contact. Hold for 5–10 seconds.
4. Repeat with opposite leg.
5. Continue for 2–4 minutes.
6. Repeat steps 1–5 with rear knee bent.

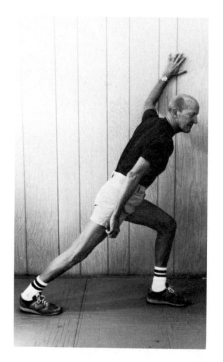

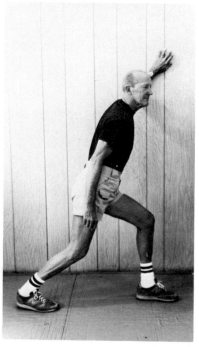

E. Barefoot jumping

1. Standing, feet as wide as shoulders, barefoot.
2. Bouncing; emphasizing heel dropping low.
3. Bounce for 30 seconds, rest for 30 seconds, repeat.
4. Continue for 2–5 minutes.

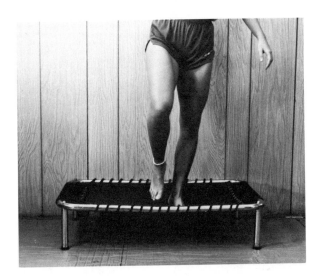

Blisters. Blisters are caused by friction between the skin and the shoe or sock. Common causes are ill-fitting or tight-fitting shoes, wrinkles in the socks, and sudden increases in the amount of exercise. Prevention of blisters can be accomplished by wearing well-fitted shoes, pulling the wrinkles out of socks, applying adhesive tape to the heels, toes or other appropriate spots and, if necessary, applying petroleum jelly to the foot before putting on the socks.

Shinsplints. The term "shinsplints" is used to describe the pain that occurs along the front or along the sides of the lower leg. Shinsplints is the result of excessive repeated walking, jogging or skating. Other causes include changing exercise shoes or switching from a soft surface to a hard surface, and it has even been said that individuals who have longer second toes (Morton's foot) may be more susceptible to stress on the front or the anterior part of the lower leg. Look at your second toe to see if it's longer than your big toe. If it is longer or if you have experienced shinsplints, the following exercises are almost guaranteed to bring relief.

F. Walk for dorsiflexion (anterior tibialis—shinsplints)

1. Standing, total weight on heels, toes lifted from floor, knees locked straight.
2. Step with short stride.
3. Walk for 50 steps, rest; repeat 5 times.
4. Repeat steps 1–3 with toes turned in.
5. Repeat steps 1–3 with toes turned out.
6. Continue for 2–5 minutes.

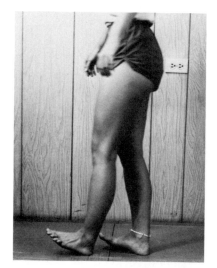
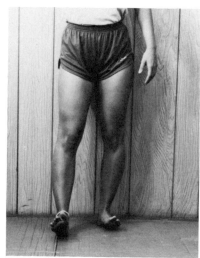
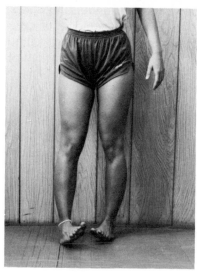
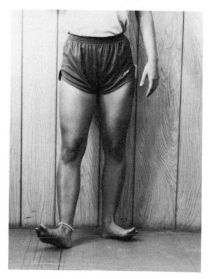

G. Walk for lateral stretch

1. Standing, barefoot, weight on sides of feet, toes curled and turned in.
2. Step with short stride.
3. Walk for 50 steps, rest; repeat 5 times.
4. Continue for 2–5 minutes.

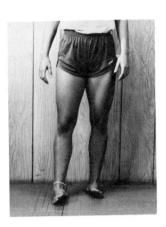

H. Lower shin stretch

1. Kneeling on floor, hands on floor.
2. Extend one leg straight back 3–4 feet with top of foot on floor.
3. Slowly bend rear knee to stretch the muscles on the lower front of the rear leg and front of the rear foot for 30 seconds.
4. Repeat using opposite leg.
5. Continue for 2–4 minutes.

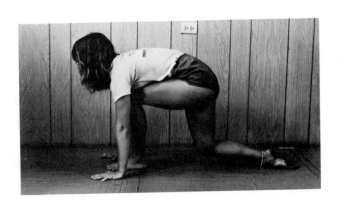

Calf pain or Achilles tendinitis.   The Achilles tendon attaches to the lower heel bone, runs up the rear of the leg and blends into the calf muscles (gastrocnemius and soleus). The calf muscle is attached at the rear lower knee. Calf pain is usually caused from exercise in which the heel is raised above the floor level, such as in stair climbing, running on the toes, toe lifts or skipping rope.

Achilles tendinitis usually occurs as a result of allowing the heel of the foot to drop down, as might happen if you were running in very soft sand or wearing shoes that have little heel padding or running in shoes with an insufficient heel counter. Achilles tendinitis can be a mild strain or a complete rupture requiring surgery. In mild Achilles tendon strains, rest and medical attention should precede rehabilitation. Avoid uphill or stair climbing during rehabilitation. In many cases, your physician or podiatrist may wish to insert a felt heel pad into both shoes to relieve the strain on the tendon.

Prevention of calf pain and Achilles tendinitis is most effectively achieved when you use the following exercises.

I. Straight ankle pull

1. Sitting position, knees bent, heels on floor, grasp toes.
2. Slowly attempt to straighten legs until reasonably straight, pull back on toes, hold for 5 seconds.
3. Return legs to bent position.
4. Continue for 1–3 minutes.

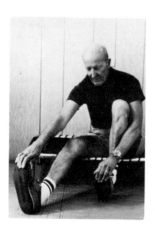
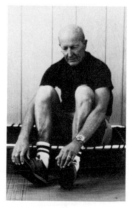
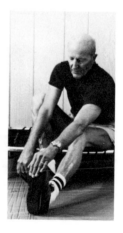

J. Lateral ankle pull

1. Sitting position, knees bent, heels on floor.
2. Grasp lateral (outside) border of foot near toes.
3. Slowly attempt to straighten legs until reasonably straight, pull back on side of foot, hold for 5 seconds.
4. Return legs to bent position.
5. Continue for 1–3 minutes.

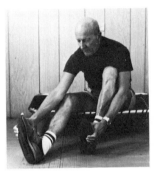 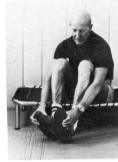 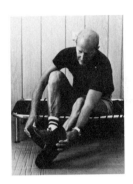

K. Medial ankle pull

1. Sitting position, knees bent, heels on floor.
2. Grasp medial (inside) border of foot, near toes.
3. Slowly attempt to straighten legs until reasonably straight, pull back on inside of foot, hold for 5 seconds.
4. Return legs to bent position.
5. Continue for 1–3 minutes.

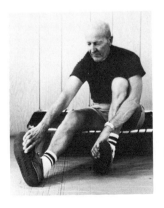 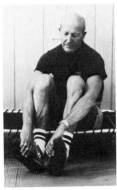 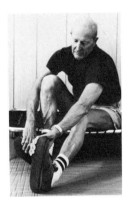

L. Achilles tendon stretch (gastrocnemius)

1. Standing 3–4 feet from wall, hands on wall.
2. Extend one leg straight back 3–4 feet with heel on floor.
3. Bend front knee and move upper body forward slowly toward wall so that rear leg muscles are stretched. Retain heel-floor contact; hold for 5 seconds.
4. Repeat using opposite leg.
5. Continue for 1–3 minutes.

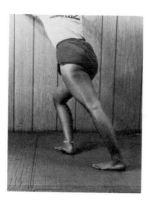

M. Achilles tendon stretch (soleus)

1. Standing 3–4 feet from wall, hands on wall.
2. Extend one leg straight back 3–4 feet with heel on floor; bend front knee and move trunk forward slowly toward wall so that rear leg muscles are stretched.
3. Slowly bend the knee of rear leg to a point of bearable pain, retaining heel-floor contact; hold for 5 seconds.
4. Repeat using opposite leg.
5. Continue for 1–3 minutes.

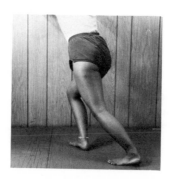

Knee injuries. The knee is the most easily damaged joint of the body. The knee joint is supported by ligaments for stability, and the strength of the knee depends greatly on the front thigh muscle and, to a lesser degree, on the rear thigh muscles. The so-called "runners knee" often results from running downhill, running with improper shoes, running barefoot, running with the toes pointed in or from suddenly increasing the amount of distance covered.

Should you develop persistent knee pain or have a knee injury, an orthopedic physician should be contacted, and the exercise that caused the knee pain should be, for the present, terminated. An alternative non-weight-bearing activity should be substituted, such as swimming or stationary bicycling. Orthotics or heel lifts may remedy acute knee pain. In most cases, jumping will not cause foot, ankle, knee, hip or back injuries. In fact, in our rehabilitation laboratory, jumping is used routinely during the rehabilitation of patients with knee joint injuries (see Appendix II, Medical Applications).

Should pain occur as a result of jumping, stop the activity and see your physician. When you start jumping again, go slowly for the first four weeks to reduce early strain.

The following exercises could be beneficial in strengthening the muscles that support the knee joint.

N. Straight leg lift

1. Sitting, one leg straight with toes pointed up, other knee bent, both elbows stable on floor or on mat.
2. Slowly raise straight leg 6 inches from floor, hold for 5 seconds, return to floor.
3. Repeat 10–20 times.
4. Repeat with other leg.
5. After preliminary strengthening, a 5- to 20-pound weight may be placed on the foot as shown in the photo.

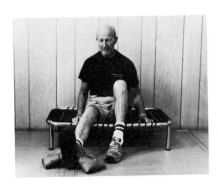 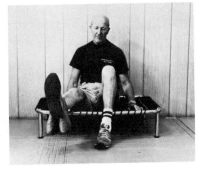

O. Sitting flutter kick

1. Sitting, both legs straight with toes pointed straight, both elbows stable on floor or mat, stomach muscles pulled in, with ankles raised 3–4 inches above floor.
2. Slowly alternate raising legs in a flutter kick.
3. Kick for 20–30 seconds, rest and repeat.
4. Flutter kick for 2–3 minutes.

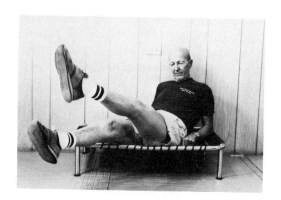

P. Stomach flutter kicks

1. Lie flat on stomach, toes extended straight.
2. Raise both legs 3–4 inches, and slowly alternate raising legs in a flutter kick.
3. Kick legs at a comfortably vigorous pace for 20–30 seconds; rest and repeat.
4. Continue for 1–3 minutes.

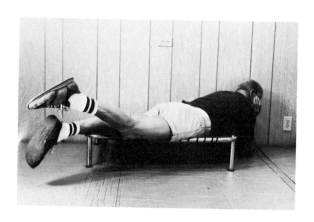

Q. Quad bounce

1. Standing on mat of rebounding equipment in ski position, feet together, poles in hand or balance with chairbacks (see Chapter 14).
2. Leave upper body still while bringing both knees up 2–6 inches. Return to mat. Repeat fairly rapidly.
3. Repeat for 15–30 seconds, stop, take a 6-second pulse count (do not exceed your exercise heart rate).
4. Continue for 3–10 minutes.

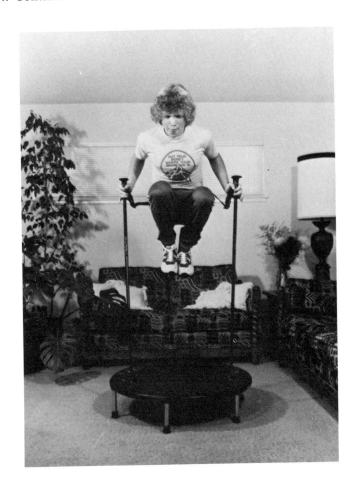

12

Eating Well—Nutrition, Cholesterol and Common Sense

Jump for Joy may be a book about exercise, but nutrition is a factor you cannot overlook. It's one of the most important ways you can improve your life-style and overall health, so this chapter is devoted to *smart eating*.

We'll go back to your risk factor test to look at your present nutritional status, and then later I'll give you some tips on how to improve your nutritional profile, how to outsmart the supermarket, how to cook cleverly and how to survive eating out.

NUTRITION*

Part E-1 of the risk factor test deals with overeating, meal-skipping and salt in the diet. Often people who overeat and are overfat experience indigestion, gastric discomfort and sleeplessness. Overeating frequently results from skipping breakfast or lunch. Skipping meals is not advisable because your blood sugar level may drop below normal levels. Many people with low blood sugar experience hypoglycemic symptoms such as irritability, shakiness, insecurity, low work productivity, shortened attention span and lack of interest.

Low blood sugar resulting from skipping meals also causes your appetite-regulating mechanism, the "appestat," to overreact. After

---

*Prepared by Melly Randolph

skipping meals all day, you sit down to a dinner and start gorging yourself, and no matter how much you eat you just don't seem to be getting that "enough feeling." So you continue eating and eating. Since it takes about 30 minutes for the appestat to register that it has received food, you have probably already overeaten.

Meal skippers report that even though they may be full of food and actually feel full, they usually have a strong desire to eat more food. This happens because the appestat has not fully recovered from skipped meals earlier in the day.

Halt, do you need salt? Probably not. We Americans eat about 10–16 grams of salt a day and really only need 1–2 grams per day. One gram is about the size of a small raisin. The way you reduce your salt intake is by not buying salty foods, such as potato chips, corn chips, nuts, sauerkraut, pickles and processed meats. Also, don't salt at the table with the salt shaker. Make a deal with yourself that you'll only lightly salt your meat and eggs. Use salt substitute and spices to add flavor to your food. Continued salt use often causes elevated blood pressure, which may result in heart disease, stroke and kidney dysfunctions.

Part E-2 looks at your caffeine intake. In coffee there is between 100 and 150 mg of caffeine; in tea, about 70 mg; in some chocolate drinks, about 50 mg; and in cola drinks, between 10 and 80 mg per drink.

Caffeine increases resting heart rate and blood pressure, has been mentioned in lay literature as an aging substance and recently has been linked strongly to breast cancer. If you decide to stop caffeine, you may experience headaches for several days.

Besides giving you a lift and appeasing your habit, we really can't find too much good about caffeine. Therefore, substituting non-caffeine drinks such as unsweetened fruit juice, herbal teas, postum or decaffeinated drinks for your present caffeine beverages is recommended.

Part E-3 checks sugar in the diet, which adds up to a hefty 125 pounds per year for every man, woman and child in this country. Sugar foods, snacks and beverages account for about 30 to 35 percent of our daily calories. Dietary sugar may elevate your normal blood sugar level of between 80 and 100 mg percent* up over 100 mg percent, sometimes as high as 130 to 150 mg percent.

High blood sugar levels cause insulin to shoot into your blood, which neutralizes the sugar by carrying it back to the liver. This is

---

*In 100 milliliters of blood, blood sugar takes up 80–100 mg, which is the measure mg percent.

nature's attempt to return your sugar level to normal. What often happens is an overreaction by the insulin, which drives the blood sugar level down below normal and guess where you are? Right back in that old hypoglycemic state.

Not only does sugar produce abnormal blood sugar levels, but it's extremely fattening, causes tooth decay and has not one vitamin. Since sugar has no vitamins and requires Vitamin B to be digested, it must strip Vitamin B from the central nervous system, thus reducing the stability of your emotional state. If you desire sweet foods try to select fresh, natural fruit.

Part E-4 concerns roughage intake in the American diet, which is low, resulting in constipation, diverticulosis, hemorrhoids and bowel cancer. Eating more whole grain cereals and raw vegetables and adding a couple of teaspoons of bran to the daily menu should relieve and reduce the digestive problems that result from too much processed food and meat in the diet.

Part E-5 is about fat. Forty-five percent of the average American's daily calories is digestible fat. That amount should be reduced to approximately 20 percent of the diet. Excess fats cause overweight, high blood pressure, increased incidence of diabetes and cancer as well as heart disease.

Saturated fats (animal fats) in the diet stimulate the liver to produce cholesterol, low-density lipoprotein (LDL), high-density lipoprotein (HDL) and triglycerides. LDL apparently can carry cholesterol throughout the arteries, where it can be deposited, causing vascular and heart disease. HDL, on the other hand, seems to protect against heart disease, probably by carrying cholesterol back to the liver, where it's metabolized. The object of the game is to get as much HDL-type cholesterol as possible and reduce the total cholesterol and LDL-type cholesterol. How do you do that?

There are several ways. They include doing daily vigorous exercise, eating limited amounts of fat, especially the saturated fats, staying away from tobacco smoke, eating extra bran and pectin in the diet each day and being as thin as is reasonable.

One last way to improve your HDL score is by drinking no more than two drinks of alcohol per day (2–3 ounces). One to two drinks tend to increase the HDL in the blood, while drinking more than two drinks per day tends to decrease the HDL.

What are saturated fats and how can we avoid them? Saturated fats are found in whole milk products, ice cream, most fat cheeses, lard, butter, egg yolks, fat meats such as pork, beef, duck, hamburger and steak, and in some vegetable oils, such as palm and coconut oil.

You can decrease your intake by eating non-fat dairy products;

reducing your total meat and cheese consumption by eating no more than a total of 3 to 4 ounces per day; limiting the amount of butter to one or two pats per day; eating fewer than five eggs per week and cooking them in water instead of butter, oil or bacon grease; eating more chicken, fish, seafood, veal and turkey (and remember to remove the skin and fat before you cook them). Meat substitutes such as beans and rice are an excellent way to get protein without animal fat.

Should you occasionally fall prey to fat-containing ice cream, cake or cherries jubilee try to take only a bite or two for the satisfaction and yield to the temptation only once or twice a month.

HOW TO EAT WELL

There are many fad diets, all claiming to be the answer to America's weight problem. What it all boils down to is that there are only a few items that you need to know in order to eat properly and still maintain your desirable weight. First, you have to learn how to buy the right foods in the market; second, how to prepare foods at home and make meals healthful; and third, how to order from a menu in a restaurant.

MARKET SHOPPING

When you enter the supermarket, consider this procedure. Wheel your shopping cart directly to the fruit and vegetable sections. Select no fewer than five different kinds of vegetables and at least three different kinds of fruits. Then wheel over to the dried-vegetable section and pick up some beans, brown rice and dried peas. Head your cart for the meat department. Purchase the smallest servings of fish, chicken, seafood, veal, very lean pork and possibly a little beef. Read the label for weight and inspect the contents to determine how many ounces of edible meat are in the package. Select a package that will provide no more than 4 ounces of meat per person.

Now head for the dairy section. Pick up a dozen fresh eggs and lots of non-fat milk, a little low-fat cheese, plain low-fat yogurt, low-fat cottage cheese and a small amount of butter if you must.

Finally, wheel your cart over to the bread section and select only whole wheat or whole grain breads. Ease down to the cereal aisle and select only whole grain, unsugared cereals such as shredded wheat and oatmeal.

While you're at the check-out counter, look at the shopping carts around you. You will probably see carts filled with whole milk, white bread, hamburger, bacon, processed foods, donuts, sugared cereals, ice cream, heavy-fat cheeses, sugary soft drinks for the kids and a single diet soda for the overweight person pushing the cart.

PREPARING FOOD AT HOME

Now that you've escaped from the supermarket without succumbing to all the advertising tricks designed to make you purchase processed, convenient and dangerous food, don't blow it when you get home. Some pertinent ideas follow.

1. Lightly steam your vegetables or sprinkle a light oil and vinegar salad dressing over your raw vegetables.
2. Bake, broil or boil your meat, and trim away any skin and fat before cooking. Season with herbs and spices but go light on the salt.
3. Avoid scrambling or frying eggs in butter, bacon grease or oil. Poached or boiled eggs are best for you.
4. Toast or heat bread, but use little or no butter or margarine.
5. For dessert, always have a little fresh fruit, or blend up a smoothie or prepare a fruit compote.

TABLE 12.1. TYPICAL MEALS AT HOME

Typical Breakfast	*Proper Breakfast*
Bacon Eggs	One egg or whole grain cereal (hot or cold)
White toast	1 slice whole wheat toast
Butter	$\frac{1}{2}$ pat butter
Jam or jelly	Citrus fruit
Whole milk	Skim milk (8 oz)
Coffee, sugar, cream or dairy creamer	Decaffeinated coffee if you must

Typical Lunch	*Proper Lunch*
Hamburger or Roast beef sandwich French fries or Mashed potatoes and gravy	$\frac{1}{2}$ sandwich Whole wheat bread Tuna, chicken, turkey or Low-Fat cheese
Well-cooked vegetables	2–3 Vegetables (celery, tomato, carrots, etc.)
Pie or ice cream	1 piece fruit
Coffee, cream and sugar	Skim milk (8 oz)

Typical Dinner	*Proper Dinner*
Salad with dressing (Blue Cheese, Sour Cream, Thousand Island or Russian)	Large green salad with salad dressing (light vinegar and oil or plain lemon juice)
Prime rib Pork chops Rack of lamb Hamburger Steak Seafood dipped in butter Breaded fried meat	Small (3 to 4 oz) serving of meat (Turkey, fish, chicken, seafood without butter, lean veal or possibly small filet mignon)
2 well-done vegetables	2–3 lightly steamed vegetables 1 small baked potato (1 pat of butter or 2 tsp sour cream or better yet 4 to 5 tbs of skim milk and whip the baked potato into a smooth, tasty, moist consistency)
White rolls or White bread and butter	1 slice whole wheat bread $\frac{1}{2}$ pat butter
Ice cream, pie, cake or other sweet, processed desserts	Fresh fruit
Whole milk	Skim milk (8 oz)
Coffee, cream and sugar	

DINING OUT—
HOW TO SURVIVE

Eating out is a treat, but there are times we tend to go overboard. We end up ordering more than we should and getting less nutrition. When you're handed the menu, read it very carefully—as though your life depended upon it. It very well may. Some hints follow.

1. When ordering an appetizer, try to select one that is of vegetable origin or that comes in it's natural state and is not fried, sautéed, or prepared with oil or heavy cheeses.
2. Order a large salad, but the salad dressing is the most important part of the order. Avoid creamed salad dressings. A couple of ladles of salad dressing can take a 100-calorie salad and bring it up to the 600- to 700-calorie range.
3. Select a vegetable soup or a clear broth instead of a cream chowder or meat soup.
4. For the entrée, select chicken, turkey, seafood or fish, lean veal or a small filet mignon. In most cases, the meat portion will be too large; try to eat only half the meat served. Remember, you can order an extra salad, one meal, and split it with your date. Probably not too impressive, but healthier.
5. Don't be afraid to order a baked potato; just don't put very much butter or sour cream on it. Two pats of butter at 85 calories each doubles a baked potato's calories. However, you can put twice the amount of sour cream as butter and get the same number of calories.
6. Limit the amount of bread you eat all the way through the meal. We tend to eat and eat whatever is placed before us.
7. For dessert try to select fresh fruit, and if that's not available, share a dessert with one or two other people. Then stop eating for the rest of the evening! In most cases, being overweight is the result of wolfing down too many calories and not exercising.

If you follow the nutritional program given above, eat three comfortable meals a day and reduce the portion size, you will not have to deprive yourself of anything because you will have your eating under control.

The calories from extra snack and junk food really add up. Americans eat about 300 calories of junk food or unnecessary food each day. Remember, 300 calories less in junk food plus 300 calories expended in exercise (30 minutes) totals 600 calories each day, and that equals one pound of fat per week that disappears from your body.

TABLE 12.2. CALORIC EQUIVALENCIES OF CERTAIN FOODS AND AMOUNT OF EXERCISE REQUIRED TO BURN OFF

Calories =	Typical Food =	Healthier Food =	Exercise to Burn Off
100	1 drink of alcohol: 4 oz wine or glass of beer or snifter of brandy	2 small apples or 1 banana or 3 oz canned shrimp	1 mile walking or jogging; 10–12 min "Jumping for Joy"
230	1 Baskin Robbins ice cream cone	1.5 lbs of carrots	25 min of slow swimming
400	3 oz candy bar	4.5 grapefruit or 10 tomatoes or 101 green olives	40 min "Jumping for Joy"
450	1 Big Mac hamburger	3 oz baked fish (or turkey or veal) + baked potato + 2 vegetables + salad + $\frac{1}{4}$ cantaloupe + glass skim milk	4.5 miles walking or jogging

TABLE 12.2. (Continued)

Calories	=	Typical Food	=	Healthier Food	=	Exercise to Burn Off
900		8 oz prime rib (usual cut is 10–16 oz)		4 oz chicken or fish (skin and fat removed); + 3 servings vegetables + salad + $\frac{1}{2}$ cup rice + whole wheat roll with pat butter + glass skim milk + fruit & lowfat yogurt		9 miles walking or jogging

WEIGHT CONTROL SCHEDULE

The following chart can be cut out and taped on the wall near your scale so that you can track your monthly weight improvement. If you follow the program faithfully, you will have all the success you need.

TABLE 12.3. JUMP FOR JOY WEIGHT CONTROL SCHEDULE

This is a monthly weight control schedule to assure you that your weight continues to tumble down.

To make it work:

Enter your present weight	(a) _____
Enter your optimal weight	(b) _____
Subtract (b) from (a)	_____

This number is the number of pounds you are going to lose over the next several months.

We want you to lose between 3 and 5 pounds of fat each month. So, enter your current weight next to the present month of the year.

Then go down the chart month by month, subtracting 4 pounds at a time and entering each month's target weight until you reach your optimal weight. For example, if you start in November, 1983, weighing 140 pounds and your optimal weight is 120 pounds, enter 136 under December, 132 under January 1984, and so on until June, 1984. This kind of slow weight loss is the easiest to accomplish and the healthiest and most long-lasting.

Month	1983	1984	1985	1986	1987
January					
February					
March					
April					
May					
June					
July					
August					
September					
October					
November					
December					

13

Especially for Women

Women in all walks of life are expressing their decision-making pow-
ers in an assertive, confident manner. Fortunately, this decisiveness
carries over to health and fitness areas as well.

Women are at a disadvantage in athletics because the absolute
work performance of men exceeds that of women by 20 percent or
more. The reasons for the differences in performance is due to the
woman's smaller body, smaller muscle size resulting in less strength
and a greater percentage of body fat than a man.

The reasons for the strength and speed differences between men
and women lie basically in the fact that the muscle mass in men may
exceed the muscle mass in women by between 30 to 50 percent. The
difference in muscle size is related to the fact that men have higher
levels of anabolic hormones (testosterone), which promote development of muscle bulk and strength.

There are several factors that can explain the woman's disadvantage in athletics in that they have smaller hearts per body mass,
have fewer red blood cells, lower hemoglobin level and smaller lung
volumes than males. Another interesting phenomenon is that the
male sex hormone, testosterone, not only enables the male to increase
his muscle mass, but also has a relationship to the response to endurance training. The male also has the advantage in that his body can
cool itself more effectively; in the female, the hormone estrogen
tends to inhibit the production of sweat. Furthermore, estrogen,
which keeps women's muscles smaller and a little bit less strong, has
been shown to have a significantly higher protective role in the development of cardiovascular disease. It probably keeps your blood cholesterol levels lower, which in the long run is more important than
being able to sweat a lot or to run the 100-yard dash in less than ten
seconds.

Remember, the incidence of heart disease is about five times higher for men than it is for women. The male, with his superior physical strength, almost uniformly suffers from elevated cholesterol, elevated blood pressure and an elevated waist line.

EXERCISE DURING MENSTRUATION

For most women, menstruation lasts for several days each month. With the discomfort and weakness that often accompanies menstruation, the question of whether or not to participate in exercise during this time needs to be discussed.

Many women claim that during their menstrual cycle they are more fatigued and tend to become lethargic. Although there is discomfort during the menstrual period, most of the research conducted has shown that this time does not adversely affect submaximal performance in the female. However, there are studies that show that as many as 50 percent of the women athletes tested perform at a lower level during menstruation. Loss of menstrual blood and subsequent reduction in red blood cells necessary to deliver oxygen to the muscle tissue may be one of the physiological reasons for the poor performance.

During menstruation, 1 to 5 ounces of blood are lost. [The blood is replaced with new blood cells formed in the bone marrow and is restored within several days after onset. During this time the number of red blood cells available to carry oxygen to the muscle tissue is reduced and a feeling of weakness may result.]

During menstruation, many women experience a variety of symptoms, including abdominal pains, which are often accompanied by water retention, abdominal swelling, nausea, backache and frequently severe headaches. Menstrual discomfort, according to Drs. Ellen Kelly, Barbara Drinkwater and others at the University of California at Santa Barbara who have conducted gynecological surveys of female athletes, is due to faulty living habits, among which are overeating, improper nutrition, tension, poor posture and a lack of exercise. Loss of strength in abdominal and back muscles probably contributes to excessively painful menstrual periods.

A recent study shows that women who have strong abdominal and back muscles have fewer abnormal and painful menstrual periods. The abdominal exercises described in Chapter 9 will increase abdominal strength and, if the relationship holds true, should reduce painful menstrual periods.

It appears that in the majority of cases and in the absence of pathology, it is both physiologically and psychologically beneficial for women to continue to exercise during menstruation. According to the *Physical Fitness Research Digest*, published by the President's Council on Physical Fitness and Sports, "Women scoring high on a bicycle ergometer test had fewer menstrual complaints than women scoring low on the test." It is therefore possible for women to participate in all exercise activities that they would have normally completed during the nonmenstrual period. Should exercising cause undue pain, discontinue that particular exercise until the completion of the menstrual period.

PREGNANCY AND EXERCISE

Most physicians now recommend that pregnant women exercise on a daily basis. It has been our observation that pregnant women who maintain a vigorous daily exercise program have relatively few difficulties before, during and after delivery. We have observed women in their sixth month running half-marathons and women in their fifth month participating in rebounding exercises.

Exercises during pregnancy should be coordinated with your physician and should be maintained at a comfortable pace. The activities recommended are brisk walking, stationary bicycling and swimming. Only recently have long-distance running and rebounding exercises been considered a form of exercise for expectant mothers. Before undertaking any kind of exercise program, ask your physician's advice.

SPECIAL CONSIDERATIONS

Jogging bra. Jumping is one activity that is so much fun that you will probably continue it for a lifetime. If you are beyond the training-bra size, I suggest you go to a jogging supply store or sports store and purchase a jogging bra. The jogging bra has extra support material and stitching to keep it intact and you comfortable.

Extra exercise. Because you are a woman, you have more fat cells than a man, and they're greater in size. Women have a lower metabolic rate and tend to conserve calories, all of which results in a greater storage of body fat.

How are you going to handle this? By exercising five, six, or even seven days a week, by progressively increasing the number of minutes you exercise week by week, and by being willing to jump in the morning and occasionally in the evening as well.

One more idea might be to jump seven days a week and also frequently perform some other type of exercise, such as bicycling, dancing, aerobic dancing or skating.

Bladder tickles. Nearly half the women in our jumping program reported that during the first few weeks, they felt the need to urinate frequently. We did a study and found that if women urinated before they exercised, the sensation was reduced. And it wasn't long before they were able to control the sensation completely.

After consulting with urologists at our local hospitals, we found that in many women the pubococcygeal, or PC, muscle—the muscle that controls the bladder—is weakened because of a lack of exercise. The urologists felt that jumping might strengthen the PC muscle and thus reduce the discomfort.

Sexual response. About 25 percent of the women who followed the jumping program for several months claimed that the exercise increased their sexual desire. We have not investigated to see if other sports activities cause increased arousal. However, it has been suggested by two sexologists at our university that increasing the strength of the PC muscle combined with any hormonal response elicited from the exercise possibly could account for increased sexual desire. This subject needs additional specific research and documentation.

14

Getting Ready for the Ski Season

If you're a downhill skier and want to know how to improve your skiing, or at least get yourself into better ski condition, this chapter will get your body ready to "go for it." This program will strengthen the muscles involved in skiing so that when you get on the hill, especially during the early part of the skiing season, you will not fatigue as you have in the past.

The ski exercises are designed to allow you to actually wear your ski boots during the stretching, the warm-up, and during the conditioning phase. We suggest that you wear your ski boots while jumping, provided the contact of your boots to the mat is not slippery or dangerous. If it is, instead of your ski boots, wear a pair of rubber-soled gym shoes or other shoes that provide proper and safe traction. Also, do not wear your ski boots on the rebounding equipment if the boots have metal attachments or other sharp parts. The mat of your mini-jumper is not designed to withstand contact with sharp metal.

If you're able to wear your boots, jumping will allow your feet and ankles to become accustomed to the flow material lining the inside of the boot, thus minimizing the "hot spots" that occur on your feet and the abrasion on the front of your shins. If you haven't broken in your boots, these painful spots almost always occur early in the season.

The 40-day pre-ski season workout will certainly improve your skiing and minimize those unnecessary pains. The exercises are designed to strengthen the muscles used in skiing. These are:

1. The quadriceps muscles support the knees and hips, and are located on the front of the upper thighs.

2. The anterior muscles of the lower legs, which support the ankles and are important for stability.
3. The muscles that support the arch, feet and toes also need to be strengthened to reduce foot pain and resist the pressure of the boots' buckling system.
4. Since you will also be using your ski poles during the training, your arms, hands and grip will be strengthened.

SKI DRILLS

The advance ski drills were designed to mimic the actual downhill turning techniques. The following instructions and photographs will allow you to strengthen the muscles used in downhill skiing.

A. Beginner wedge The feet are placed as wide as the shoulders, the lower arms are parallel to the floor. A simple double-foot bounce is used, with both feet striking the mat at the same time. The weight is placed on the inside of the feet. The shoulders face straight ahead, and with each bounce the body rotates slightly to the right, continues as far as is comfortable, and then rotates to the left so that turning slowly is practiced.

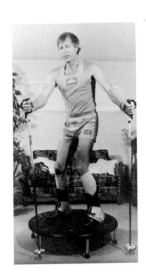
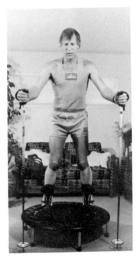
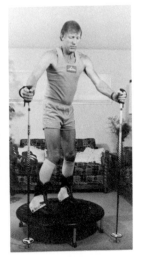

B. Intermediate parallel The feet are held 4–6 inches apart, the lower arms are parallel to the floor and the hands hold the ski poles. With the shoulders facing straight ahead, the hips are swung from side to side. The total swing covers about 12 inches of distance. Note that the upper body does not move either up and down or from side to side.

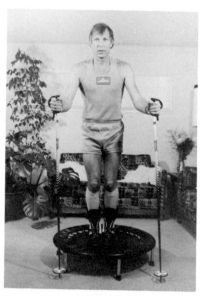

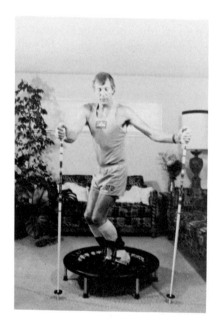

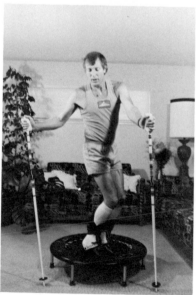

C. Advance parallel Feet are placed within 2 inches of one another, the shoulders are level, the lower arms are parallel to the floor and the hands hold the ski poles. With the upper body perfectly still, the hips are swung from side to side. The distance covered is greater than 12 inches and depends on the individual's hip flexibility and balancing skill.

For those who wish to practice extreme parallel skiing, place the boots, calves, knees and thighs firmly together. Maintain that firm contact during the parallel swings. If you're "hard core," you may place a wallet between your knees. If it falls during your workout, you lose.

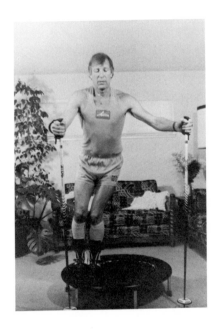

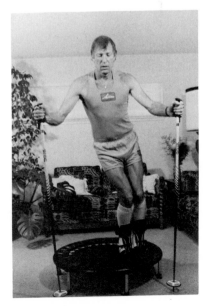

D. Quad strengthening on toes   Toe raising is an effective way of strengthening the quadriceps and conditioning the ankles and feet to the contour of the interior lining of the boot. Toe raising is exactly like quadriceps strengthening except that the toes don't leave the mat or floor. The knees bend and your waistline drops as in the "down unweighting" maneuver.

1. Standing in upright position, poles in hand, feet flat on floor.
2. Simultaneously raise up on toes and drop hips.
3. Hold for 5–15 seconds.
4. Return to standing position, feet flat.
5. Repeat one to four times for a total of 3–5 minutes.

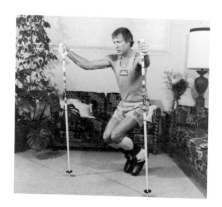

E. Quad strengthener   Since the quadriceps tend to fatigue and cause a burning sensation on long downhill treks, it is crucial that they be maximally strengthened. For this drill, you have to imagine that you are sitting in a chair with your feet on the floor. Without moving any part of your body, simultaneously lift both feet from the mat, replace them quickly, and repeat for about 5–10 seconds. From the knees up, the body is motionless and facing forward. All work is done by lifting the feet from the mat and raising the knees about 3 inches.

Once you've mastered the quad drill, you will probably gain the most benefit if you do 30 seconds of rapid quad bouncing, followed by 30 seconds of slow recovery bouncing, followed by 30 seconds of rapid quad bouncing, etc.

Usually 10 to 20 repetitions of quad jumping is considered a very good workout. The higher you bring your knees, the greater the intensity of training. Monitor your pulse so that you will not exceed your exercise heart rate.

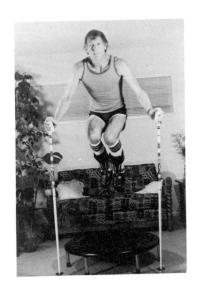

F. Mogul jumps (advanced skiers)   To get ready for the bumps, the high and low mogul jumps should be practiced. After a minute or two of advanced parallel skiing, bend the knees and hips more vigorously to the side, then return to the mat and continue parallel jumping.

Very advanced jumpers can practice a single bounce, followed by a mogul jump to the right, followed by a single bounce, followed by a mogul jump to the left.

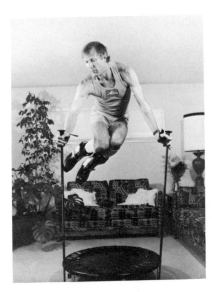
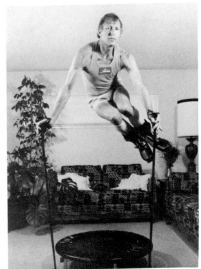

G. Skipping rope   Rope skipping is an excellent method of strengthening the quadriceps and practicing ski bouncing. You will notice that it is nearly impossible to do very rapid rope skipping on rebounding equipment. Should you want to do more rapid skipping, you might try it on your carpet or on grass, but beware: skipping rope often results in shinsplints and other leg problems when practiced on hard surfaces.

H. Single-leg parallel (advanced skiers)   Maintain the parallel position, but bring one boot 3 inches above the mat and press it lightly to the opposite boot. Parallel bounce from side to side until somewhat fatigued. Alternate to the opposite side. Advanced skiers may continue single-leg parallel exercise for 5–30 minutes for maximal strengthening.

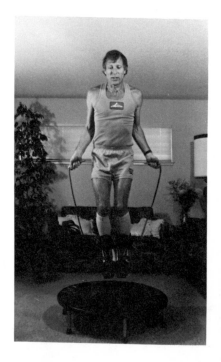

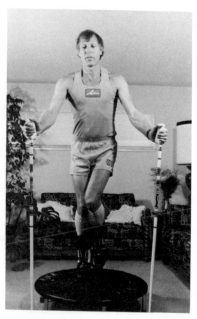

ARM EXERCISES

Your ski activities should be vigorous enough to achieve your exercise heart rate. Then, during cool-down, go for five to ten minutes of slow parallel bouncing. During the cool-down you may wish to use your ski poles to develop additional strength in the shoulders, arms and grip muscles.

I. Cymbals While parallel jumping, hold poles by the midshaft, at shoulder height, then bring them together in front of body, return to the side, return to the front, etc. The same drill can be accomplished by holding the handle of the poles.

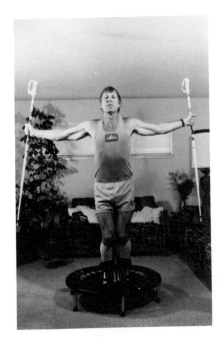

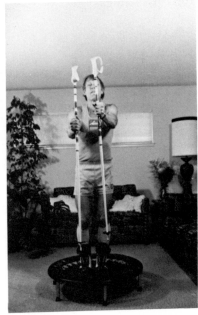

J. Propeller　Grasping the middle of both poles, rotate in a clockwise manner, then quickly rotate in a counterclockwise manner, etc. The poles also may be held overhead to achieve the propeller drill.

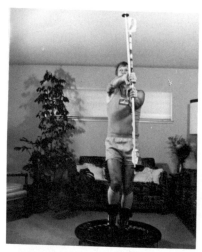
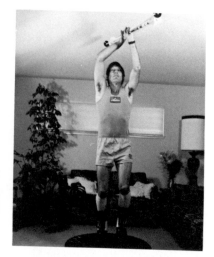

K. Hand over hand　Holding the middle of the poles to the extreme side, bring the poles to the opposite side and, as you do, give a half-turn so that the handles are now in a down position. Repeat for 1–2 minutes.

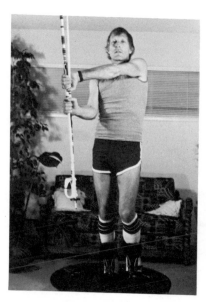
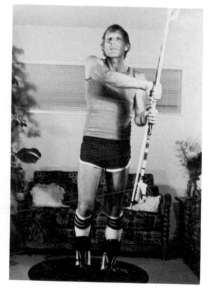

L. Swing overhead Holding the middle of the poles just above the knees, swing them to above your head, return to knees, etc.

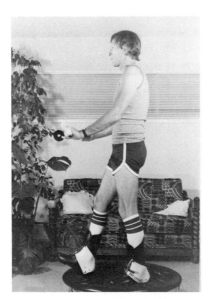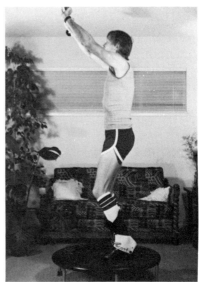

M. Ninety degree (90°) twist Keeping the knees and feet straight ahead, rotate the shoulders and ski poles to 45° to the right, then 45° to the left, etc.

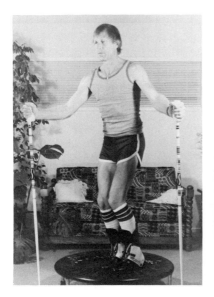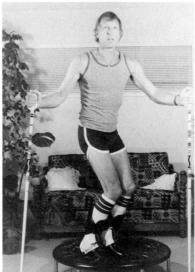

A DAILY PROGRAM TO GET READY FOR SKIING

When you arrive at your favorite ski resort, we want you to be so well conditioned that you'll be able to ski all day with maximum enjoyment. We have a six-week pre-ski season tune-up plan guaranteed to strengthen your skiing muscles so you can master the more difficult runs.

This pre-ski season training schedule is based on the assumption that you are currently exercising and are in the "high fitness" category (see pages 54–56). If you have been inactive, you should follow the program outlined in Chapter 9 for seven to ten weeks before attempting the more vigorous ski training program outlined here. Sorry, but there aren't any shortcuts!

Ski training carries you to jumping intensities ranging between 75 to 85 percent of your maximum effort, and you maintain that level for 15 to 30 continuous minutes.

To determine your ski training heart rate, locate your age and sex on Table 14.1 or 14.2 below, and read the heart rate per six-second count.

TABLE 14.1. SKI TRAINING HEART RATE FOR WOMEN

Age	Training Heart Rate (per 6 sec)	Warm-up/Cool-down Heart Rate (per 6 sec)
12–18	17–19	14–16
19–25	16–18	14–15
26–33	16–18	13–15
34–41	16–17	13–14
42–48	15–17	12–14
49–55	14–16	12–13
56–63	13–15	11–13
64–69	13–15	11–12
70+	12–14	10–12

TABLE 14.2. SKI TRAINING HEART RATE FOR MEN

Age	Training Heart Rate (per 6 sec)	Warm-up/Cool-down Heart Rate (per 6 sec)
12–18	17–18	14–15
19–25	16–17	13–14
26–33	16–17	13–14
34–41	15–16	12–13
42–48	14–15	11–12
49–55	14–15	11–12
56–63	13–14	10–11
64–69	13–14	10–11
70+	12–13	10–11

Now that you know your ski training heart rate, Table 14.3 will guide your workouts for strength and stamina.

Here's how it works. Suppose you're a 45-year-old, well-conditioned male skier preparing for a week of downhill skiing. First, from Table 14.2 you determine that your training heart rate is 14–15 beats per six-second count. At the same time, you find that your warm-up and cool-down heart rate is 11–12 beats per six seconds.

Looking at the six-week workout schedule above, you find that you should put on your boots, grab your ski poles and warm up for five minutes of light jumping and easy "parallel skiing" at an intensity that will get your heart rate up to 11–12 beats per six seconds. Next is 12 minutes of parallel skiing, followed by one minute of rope skipping. To fully strengthen your upper thighs, grab your ski poles and do ten repetitions of 15 seconds of quad jumps, followed by 30 seconds of easy recovery. After that, perform five mogul jumps on each side and, for the last exercise, 30 seconds of single-leg jumps on each foot. Five to ten minutes of slow jumping as a cool-down finishes the session. You can do your arm exercises during the cool-down.

As you can see from the schedule, the second week is slightly more vigorous. By the sixth week, you'll be in top shape for the best turns of your life.

TABLE 14.3.   PRE-SKI SEASON WORKOUTS*
(FOUR TO FIVE DAYS PER WEEK)

Week	Warm-up	Ski Parallel (P. 161)	Skip Rope (P. 166)	Quad Strengthening (P. 164)	Moguls (P. 165)	Single-leg Parallel Drill (P. 166)	Cool-down Arm Exercises
1	5 min	12 min	1 min	REPEAT 10 TIMES 15 sec. exer./30 sec. rest	5 each side	30 sec. each foot	5–10 min
2	→	15 min	2 min	REPEAT 10 TIMES 20 sec. exer./30 sec. rest	5 each side	60 sec. each foot	→
3	→	18 min	3 min	REPEAT 12 TIMES 20 sec. exer./30 sec. rest	7 each side	2 min each foot	→
4	→	21 min	4 min	REPEAT 15 TIMES 25 sec. exer./30 sec. rest	8 each side	3 min each foot	
5	→	25 min	5 min	REPEAT 15 TIMES 27 sec. exer./30 sec. rest	9 each side	4 min each foot	→
6	→	30 min +	6 min	REPEAT 15 TIMES 30 sec. exer./30 sec. rest	10 each side	5 min each foot	→

*Monitor your heart rate often. It's not advisable to exceed your established exercise heart rate.

STRENGTHENING AND STRETCHING EXERCISES

Utilizing Your Ski Equipment

To be performed on a carpeted floor, wearing your socks, ski boots, ski poles and skis, before you stretch or strengthen your ski muscles. Follow the exercises with slow non-jerky movements.

N. Ankle circles (360°)

1. Standing on floor in ski position.
2. Simultaneously rotate knees in clockwise rotation for ten seconds.
3. Repeat in counterclockwise rotation for 10 seconds.
4. Repeat for 1–2 minutes.

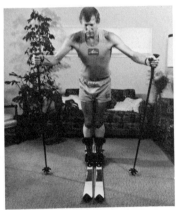
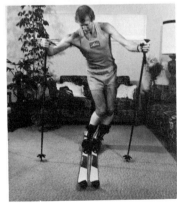
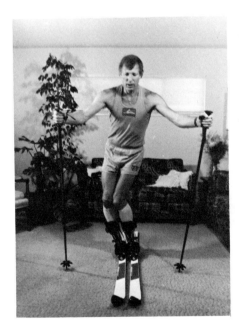

O. One step ahead

1. Standing on floor.
2. Slide skis past each other to stretch rear leg.
3. Continue for 10–20 seconds, rest and repeat with other leg.
4. Repeat for 1–2 minutes.

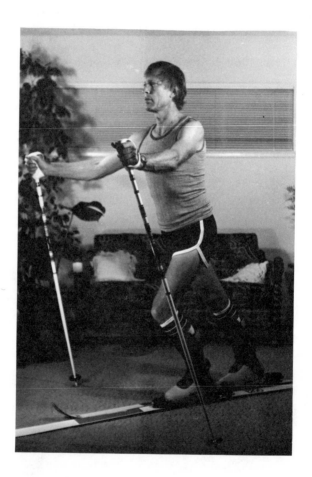

P. Tip and tail

1. Standing in ski position.
2. Lift one ski 12 inches and alternately touch tip and then tail of ski to floor.
3. Continue for 20 seconds, rest and repeat with opposite leg.
4. Repeat for 1–2 minutes.

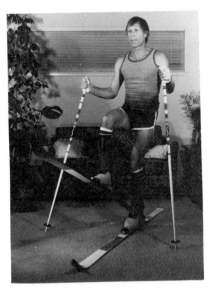
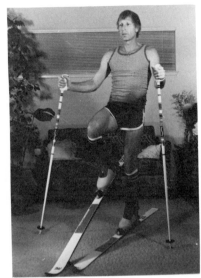

Q. Front lean

1. Standing, legs straight.
2. Slowly bend forward keeping moderate pressure on front of ski boot; hold for 5 seconds.
3. Return to standing and repeat.
4. Repeat for 1 minute.

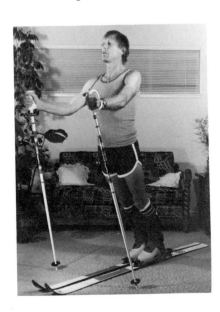
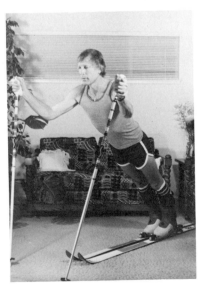

R. Side ankle stretch

1. Knees and feet straight ahead, shoulders and arms level.
2. Lean the knees out to the right and stretch the outside of the ankle and lower leg; hold for 5–15 seconds.
3. Repeat to the opposite side.
4. Continue for 1–2 minutes.

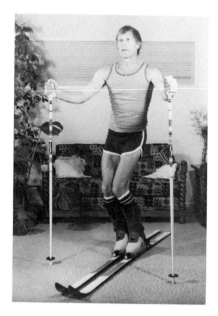

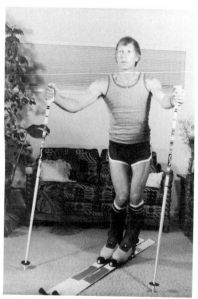

S. Sitback

1. Standing, legs straight.
2. Slowly bend knees and approximate a sitting position; hold for 5 seconds. (Do not sit lower than you would in a straight-back chair.)
3. Return to standing, rest and repeat.
4. Repeat for 2 minutes.

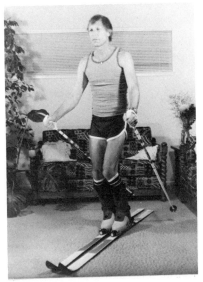

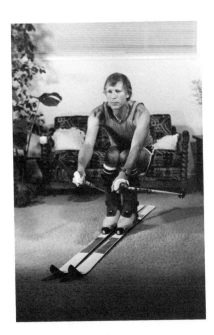

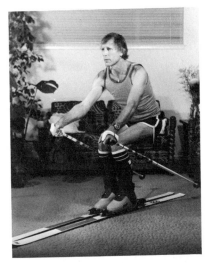

T. Slow twist

1. Standing in ski position.
2. Slowly "do the twist" for 30 seconds.
3. Rest and repeat for 1–2 minutes.

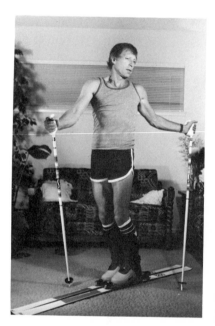

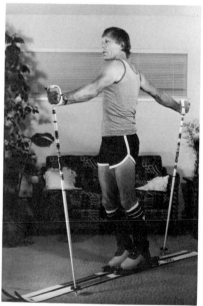

U. Side stretch (upper body)

1. Standing in ski position.
2. Extend right hip to side, weight on right ski (form a "C" shape with body); hold for 5–10 seconds.
3. Repeat on opposite side.
4. Continue for 1–2 minutes.

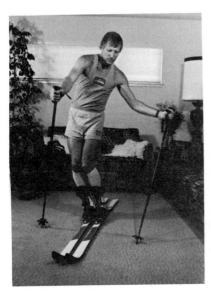 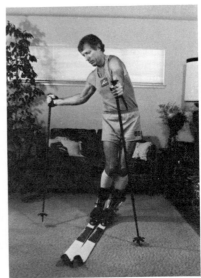

V. Wrist flick

1. Standing in ski position.
2. Alternately flick wrist to simulate pole plant for 20 seconds.
3. Rest and repeat for 1–2 minutes.

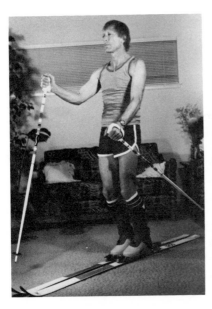 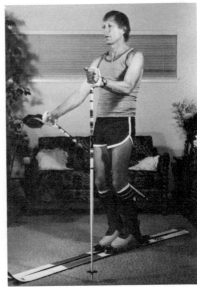

STRETCHES

The following exercises are designed to stretch and warm up healthy joints and muscles utilized in skiing. Some of the exercises are to be used on the chair lift, and others may be used before the downhill run. These exercises can be completed in five to seven minutes.

Chair-lift Exercises

(Grasp chair firmly with hands during exercises)

W. Toe curls

1. Seated in chair lift, legs dangling.
2. Flex, curl and extend toes for 20 seconds.
3. Rest for 10 seconds and repeat several times.

X. Knee

1. Seated in chair lift.
2. Alternately swing lower legs for 30 seconds.
3. Rest for 10 seconds and repeat several times.

Y. Knee lifts

1. Seated in chair lift.
2. Slowly raise one knee off the chair and hold for 5 seconds.
3. Return, rest, and repeat with opposite leg.

Z. Shoulder rotation

1. Seated in chair.
2. Elevate and rotate both shoulders for 10 seconds.
3. Rest 5 seconds and repeat several times.

ON THE MOUNTAIN— HINTS AND TIPS

1. The first runs of the day should be done slowly as a form of warm-up.
2. During the downhill run, frequent short pauses are recommended.

3. Eat early enough so that at least two hours elapse between eating and skiing.
4. Unnecessary injuries result from improper warm-up and usually occur after two to two and a half hours of continual skiing. Take a rest after two hours and be especially aware that most injuries occur during the last run or two of the day. If you are tired, call it quits for the day.
5. High altitude increases lung demand. It is best not to ski so rapidly that it causes rapid and labored breathing.
6. Drinking alcohol opens the blood vessels in the hands and feet and causes a more rapid loss of body heat. Alcohol does not warm the body. It will, after a short time, cause one to feel chilled.
7. Drinking alcohol also causes the arteries in the heart to constrict, which reduces the available blood and oxygen to the heart. This condition could be dangerous to anyone and especially those over the age of 35.
8. To keep your hands and feet from getting chilled, wear a warm cap. A great deal of body heat (30–50 percent) is lost from an uncovered head.
9. If a break for lunch is taken, it is recommended that you loosen or remove your boots. Slowly eat small portions and reduce or avoid intake of alcoholic beverages. Wait and rest for a reasonable length of time before resuming your skiing. Warm up before skiing and make the first runs slowly to stress proper form, not speed.
10. Speed jumps and fast skiing on icy moguls irritate knees. So take it easy and remember your age.

Appendices

I

Answers to the Most Commonly Asked Questions

I am only ten pounds overweight, but I really look fat. Why?

For every pound you are overweight, you are probably 2 to 4 pounds overfat. You have lost muscle and gained two to four times that weight in fat. Since fat occupies more space than muscle, you'll have that "fat look" for a few more weeks. If you continue jumping, you'll lose that look forever!

After exercising for three to four months, I seemed to get stale and felt like quitting. Is this natural?

At the beginning there is usually a great interest in exercising. As time goes by, however, it may become somewhat boring. To improve the situation, exercise with a partner and mix up the types of exercise. For example, jump three days a week, on Monday, Wednesday and Friday, and on Tuesday and Thursday you might want to go bicycling, swimming, skating, jogging or aerobic dancing. On Saturday take a one-hour walk or go dancing.

Why is it important to cool down?

Cooling down assists in removing certain acids that are formed in the muscles and blood. It also reduces soreness, stiffness and muscle cramps.

Sometimes during exercise my legs begin to hurt and occasionally, when I over-exercise, my muscles become sore. What causes this, and how can I reduce it?

Leg pain is usually a sign that you're overdoing it, either by exercising too vigorously or for too long a period of time. Increase your warm-up time and slow your pace. If this doesn't help, see your physician. You might be gouty, arthritic or have high uric acid levels.

As a large woman, I am afraid of developing large bulging muscles. Will this happen if I use weight lifting as a form of exercise?

As a woman, you have a very limited amount of testosterone in your blood. Therefore, if you lift moderately two to three days per week, you won't develop the bulging muscles that are seen on male weight lifters.

I enjoy jumping on my rebounding equipment but don't know how vigorously to exercise. Can you help?

Yes, if you jump too slowly, you will not receive the conditioning effect you want; in order to get a reasonable caloric burn-off, you would have to jump for hours. If you jump too fast, you become over-fatigued and you would only be able to last a minute or so. Look back to Chapter 8 and reestablish your exercise heart rate. Then follow the program designed in Chapter 9.

Is it really important to jump at the designated heart rate?

Yes, when you use the six-second pulse monitoring technique, it allows you to exercise at a heart rate designed to condition you properly. There is safety in not over-exercising. Jumping is fun and non-traumatic, resulting in a tendency to jump at a heart rate lower than your exercise heart rate. When you underexercise, you will not be getting the full effects to improve fitness and caloric burn-off.

Is it true that you shouldn't take your pulse with your thumb?

It's okay to use your thumb or any of your fingers to take your pulse. You will not get the so-called "double count" if you use your thumb. It's best to feel for your pulse on the wrist because using the neck could give you an inaccurate count; and in some people, pressing on the neck causes irregular heartbeats.

I read that most joggers have well-muscled legs but have thin, small muscles in the upper body. Will this happen if I jump for joy?

Long-distance runners tend to have thin upper bodies because exercise has removed the fat from the entire body. Also, most runners don't bother with upper-body exercises. When you jump, utilize vigorous arm movement because as you exercise the entire body will lose fat, but the muscles of the arms and upper body will increase and look more shapely.

I swim a lot, but can't seem to lose body fat. Is there a reason for this?

Yes, the reason that you have not lost fat on a swimming program may be because most water-living animals have an extra-thick layer of fat cells beneath the skin. When swimming in cold water, there may be a tendency for your body to pack those cells with fat in order to insulate you from the cold, thus producing the chubby appearance.

After jumping for four months I didn't lose a pound of weight, but I seemed to lose all the "cellulite." Is this normal?

When you exercise, you may or may not lose weight. You are decreasing the fat and increasing your muscle size, and this is what you want. As far as "cellulite" is concerned, there is no such thing. The word was coined by promoters. It simply describes excessive body fat that causes the skin to look dimpled. You cannot break it up or vibrate it away. The only true way to get rid of it is with daily exercise and a reasonable reduction in excess calories. The combination is the secret.

I work all day in the kitchen, do the housekeeping, and even mow the lawn. Are you going to tell me that, on top of all, I should exercise?

Not necessarily, but just look at yourself. Are you trim and happy with your body? If so, the amount of calories you are taking in is balanced with the amount of exercise you are doing around the house in the form of housekeeping. If you're like most American women, you're probably a bit overweight. If you want to lose that weight, jump four to six days per week, watch your extra calories and, if you continue for several months, you can look forward to a more girlish figure.

What is this "stitch in the side"?

We're not sure, but it could be a pain under the ribs from intestinal gas, spasms of the digestive tract, pain in the suspensory ligaments of the internal organs or a lack of blood in the diaphragm muscle. It rarely occurs when jumping on rebounding equipment, but if it does, continue jogging in place and, as you do, inhale deeply and try to stretch the abdominal muscle. After a full inhalation, fully blow the air out and bend forward as you continue jogging on the rebounding equipment. Attempt this several times and in most cases the stitch in the side will disappear. If you're a jogger, this technique also works and you don't even have to slow down while jogging.

Sometimes I get out of breath. Why does this happen?

It's happening because you are exercising at a too rapid pace. Slow your pace a bit, and remember that you should be able to carry on a conversation when you exercise. If you find yourself gasping, you're going too fast.

Will jumping improve my bones, muscles and tendons?

We think it will. Vigorous exercise should maintain normal bone strength and function as well as increase the thickness and the strength of the cartilages that protect the ends of the bones. Exercise also increases the strength of the ligaments that support the joints.

Are rubber suits, plastic suits or wraparound materials advisable?

No, in fact they're dangerous. During exercise you need to perspire to prevent overheating. When the body is covered with plastic or rubber material, the natural cooling process is inhibited and the temperatures inside your body may rise as high as 103° to 108°—certainly very dangerous temperatures. Remember, when you exercise, stay cool.

Can I profit from greater fitness?

You probably can and in more ways than one. It appears that some insurance companies now give a decrease in the annual premiums for policy holders who do not smoke and who are on exercise programs for a year or more. The premium discounts add up to a sizable 20-percent reduction because physically fit nonsmokers have a longer life expectancy than the average. The insurance companies feel that you will be able to pay an additional 12 years of premium payments if you take care of yourself.

Is there any reason to continue monitoring the pulse after exercise is finished?

Yes, you might be interested in monitoring your pulse rate after finishing your exercises because the recovery pulse rate should

return below 100 beats per minute within five minutes after you finish exercising. If the recovery pulse does not return within that time,
it may be an indication that the exercise was too vigorous for your
present fitness level.

*After we have been jumping for a while, is there another way to deter-
mine our fitness?*

Yes, by recording the postexercise heart rate you can, with some
degree of accuracy, determine your fitness level. In short, the faster
the heart rate slows after you finish exercising, the greater your fitness level. Figure A.1 will give you some idea about recovery heart
rates. Note that the well-conditioned person achieves a much lower
recovery rate much sooner than the less-fit person.

TABLE A.1.   ESTIMATION OF FITNESS FROM POSTEXERCISE RECOVERY

Heart rate difference (D)	Fitness level	Estimated $\dot{V} O_2$ max in $mlO_2/kg/min$
1 or 2	Poor	29 or less
3	Low	30–37
4	Fair	38–42
5	Good	43–50
6	Very good	51–54
7	Excellent	55–60
8 or more	Competition	61 or more

Now, to determine your fitness level from your postexercise
heart rate, first take a six-second pulse count and record your resting
heart rate at (a) below. Next, after a normal warm-up, exercise for
three to five minutes at your exercise heart rate. Stop, take an immediate six-second heart rate and record your exercise heart rate at (b).
Now sit comfortably and quietly for 60 seconds. At the end of 60 seconds, take another six-second count and record your one-minute
postexercise heart rate at (c). Finally, subtract (c) from (b) and enter
the difference at (d).

(a) _____
(b) _____
(c) _____
(d) _____

If the difference between the exercise heart rate and the recovery heart rate as depicted on line (d) is 6 or more, then you're probably in great shape. On the other hand, if the difference is 1–3, you probably need to exercise more frequently and a little more vigorously.

To estimate your fitness, compare your score recorded on line (d) with the numbers listed in column D of Table A.1. For example, if your score in line (d) is 4, then you are in fair condition and utilizing about 38 to 42 $m10_2/kg/min$.

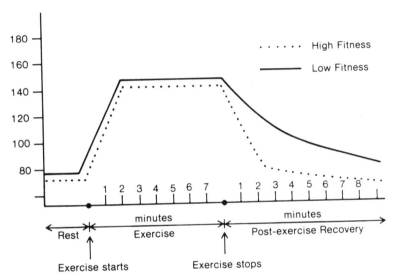

Figure A.1. Post-exercise Recovery Heart Rate Fitness Determinant.

The way to improve your fitness score is to jump nearly every day. After a few weeks, repeat the postexercise recovery test. You should be delighted by the improvement.

Do I really need to exercise four, five or six times a week?

A good rule is never to let two days go by in a row without exercising. Studies have shown that when muscles are not exercised for 48 to 72 hours, they reduce in size and strength. In fact, your muscles will reduce in size and strength in six to eight hours as you sleep overnight.

One other point, when you exercise you burn off "bad" hormones and actually produce "good" hormones. If you feel that you're emotionally stressed, you might benefit greatly from exercising six to seven days per week because that brings about greater biochemical benefits, maximizing the psychological benefits.

I read in a nutrition book that eating hamburgers and other fast-food items is really not that bad for me. Is this true?

It's true if you don't mind eating meals that are over 50 percent saturated fat, have minimal nutrients, maximal calories and are devoid of roughage. If you have to go for that fast food, limit it to two to three times a month. Your body deserves better care.

Could sex be considered a strenuous exercise?

Thought you'd never ask. Prior studies indicated that there are significant increases in pulse rate during sex and during sexual fantasies. They erroneously reported that during sexual intercourse pulse rates reach between 150 and 180 beats per minute. If this were true, sex would probably replace jogging as the number one aerobic activity in the country.

However, more recent research by Hellerstein and others have shown that peak pulse rates during sexual intercourse usually do not exceed 120 beats per minute. Sorry, but heart rates during sex fall far below the prescribed exercise heart rate, and we suspect that some may fall short of the time required to produce adequate fitness.

II

Medical Applications

Kenneth Smyth, M.D., head of the Department of Rehabilitation at Elks Hospital in Boise, Idaho, recently reported that he had successfully prescribed jumping on rebounding equipment for patients with various orthopedic and neuromuscular conditions. He asked if we had made similar clinical observations that would support his findings.

Looking over records collected in our rehabilitation lab at the University of California, San Diego, we found that we had treated over 2300 medically referred patients. Along with traditional therapy, a major factor in our rehabilitation scheme for many patients was the incorporation of jumping on rebounding equipment. For the vast majority, jumping could be used successfully. For a small minority (approximately 7 percent), jumping was contraindicated.

Jumping was used to strengthen muscles, prevent injuries, rehabilitate injuries of the lower extremities following surgery and trauma and rehabilitate and improve other medical conditions, including traumatic, osteo- and rheumatoid arthritis as well as pulmonary and cardiac disease. In short, almost any medical condition that would normally incorporate aerobic training as part of the rehabilitation process could utilize jumping as the aerobic component.

The typical postoperative knee patient would receive the following program.

1. Precast-removal exercises to strengthen the quadriceps.
2. Postcast-removal treatment (Weeks 1–3).
    a. Ice massage (8–10 minutes).
    b. Active range of motion (5–10 minutes).

   c. PNF* knee patterns.

   d. Straight leg lifts (with or without ankle weights).

3. Continued treatment (Weeks 4–6).

   a. Repeat 2a–d.

   b. Bicycle ergometer (R.O.M. friction-free). Increasing work loads according to patient response.

   c. Mini-gym (15° leg extension).

4. Continued treatment (Weeks 7–10).

   a. Continued weekly increase in repetitions and resistance for bicycling, mini-gym and leg lifts.

   b. Introduce rebounding (1–3 minutes, progressing to 30 minutes).

5. Continued treatment (Week 11 and after).

   a. Retain all appropriate treatments cited above.

   b. Introduce treadmill running if prescribed.

A tabulation of the injuries successfully treated using jumping on rebounding equipment as a portion of the total rehabilitation program is categorized below.

Foot   Painful or abnormal feet often lead to disabilities in other parts of the body. Disabilities may include bad posture, upper- and lower-back pain, headache, feelings of fatigue and frustration as well as muscular cramps.

1. *Foot strain* (acute and chronic strain) occurs in the mid-metatarsal area from an isolated incident or from use that grossly overtaxes the foot. Strain often occurs in the longitudinal arch. (See pages 133–137.)
2. *Flat feet.* (See pages 133–137.)
3. *Transverse arch* frequently occurs in women and includes pain in the instep (metatarsalgia). High-heeled shoes and weakness of the intrinsic muscle of the foot are frequently the cause.
4. *Hallux valgus, Hallus rigidus* and *hammer toe.*
5. *Osteomalacia.*
6. *Adolescent foot problems* include flattening feet, pigeon toes, congenital talipes equinovarus and congenital calcaneovalgus. (See pages 133–137.)

---

*PNF is Proprioceptive Neuromuscular Facilitation. The original work on the technique was done by Maggie Knott, and it has been more recently refined by Bob Moore, head athletic trainer at San Diego State University.

Tibia

1. *Ankle sprain* and *strain.*
2. *Anterior and posterior injuries* include shinsplints, anterior compartment pain syndrome and achilles tendon injuries. (See pages 139–142.)

Knee

1. *Patella* damage includes chondromalacia, osteochondritis dissecans/Osgood–Schlatter's disease.
2. *Ligament and cartilage damage.*
3. *Post trauma* and *post operative* rehabilitation. (See pages 143–145.)

Hip Joint and Pelvic Girdle   Injury rehabilitation may be enhanced with rebounding activities.

1. *Anterior* and *posterior femoral injuries.*
2. *Congenital degenerative mechanical abnormalities.*
3. *Degenerative arthritis.*
4. *Prosthetic replacement* (low-friction arthroplasty).

Spine, Sacrum and Coccyx   Posture defects may be improved by increasing the strength of abdominal muscles and stretching both erector spinae muscles and rear thigh muscles. (See pages 91–93.)

1. *Low back pain* resulting from improper pelvic tilt; acute back sprain; chronic back strain; intervertebral discs, ruptured disc or slipped disc.*
2. *Laminectomy.**
3. *Sciatic nerve pinch.*
4. *Schuermann's disease.**
5. *Scoliosis; degenerative arthritis of the spine.**
6. *Cervical whiplash injuries.**

---

*Usually not recommended to jump within three to six weeks following surgery. We have always requested permission from an orthopedic surgeon before initiating a jumping program. It is important to remember that the impact measured in G force on the spinal level during jumping is no greater than that measured during walking on a hardwood floor.

Other Medical Uses

1. Weight control for patients with *diabetes, hypoglycemia* and *hypertension.*
2. *Cardiac abnormalities* and *post-myocardial infarction rehabilitation.*
3. *Phlebitis.*
4. *Emotional stress* reduction as well as improvement of *depression* and *anxiety.*
5. *Chronic obstructive pulmonary disease.*
6. *Respiratory abnormalities; asthma* and *bronchitis.*
7. *Hodgkin's disease* and other *lymphatic system abnormalities.*
8. *Parkinson's disease.*
9. Various *neuromuscular abnormalities.*

The patients with the conditions listed above were referred to our laboratory from physicians practicing at the university. Jumping on rebounding equipment was one of several methods of rehabilitation and prevention, and was used as one portion of the total rehabilitation scheme. Most patients were given exercise options and were counseled on the benefits of proper nutrition and improved lifestyle habits.

Jumping on rebounding equipment is not the cure for the above conditions, but is a viable method of aerobic exercise that has a good safety record, can be controlled, is easily prescribed and is enjoyable. There were rare occasions when jumping proved not to be the best exercise for a particular individual. In those cases other forms of exercise were developed. They included swimming and/or stationary bicycling.

Our experience tells us that there are trial-and-error aspects to any exercise prescription. We feel that a cautious prescription with early and frequent appraisal of the benefits of the specific exercise will maximize results. Our physicians have found that the exercise a patient *will do*, is generally *the best* for that individual.

The preceding medical applications is intended for members of the healing arts, not lay persons. In this regard, it is recognized that rebounding equipment is sold only for exercise purposes by the various firms manufacturing such equipment, and it should also be noted that any medical applications involving use of rebounding equipment should be made only by medical prescription and direction, according to the individual judgment of the practitioner.

III

Glossary

Acclimatization. Physiological and psychological adjustment following exposure to changes in climate, humidity and altitude.

Acute. An occurrence or condition that comes on quickly.

Adipose tissue. Fat that has accumulated in the "fat cells" beneath the skin and throughout the body.

Adrenaline (epinephrine). A chemical hormone produced in the adrenal medulla and sympathetic nerve endings. When liberated, it increases the heart rate, blood pressure and hand tremor and alerts you for physical and mental action.

Agility. Ability to move quickly and change direction rapidly and smoothly while maintaining control of the body.

Aerobic exercise. Prolonged exercise during which the amount of oxygen needed by the working muscles is delivered through active breathing. The exercise heart rate is based on this principle.

Aerobic fitness (VO$_2$ max). The maximum amount of oxygen your muscles can consume for every kilogram of body weight during the last minute of maximal exercise. It is also known as oxygen uptake or maximal oxygen consumption.

Altitude sickness. The feeling of illness resulting from reduced oxygen pressure at high altitudes. Symptoms include loss of appetite, headache, rapid heart rate, rapid breathing, nausea and even vomiting.

Amino acids. The "alphabet" of protein structure. There are 22 amino acids, and all the proteins in our bodies are made up of amino acids in combinations ranging in number from a few to many thousands.

Anaerobic exercise.   Exercises defined by intense activity of short duration, after which a rest is needed with fairly heavy breathing in order to pay back the "oxygen debt" that occurred during the exercise. Anaerobic exercises are sprinting, racquetball, singles tennis, etc.

Androgen (testosterone).   Male sex hormone manufactured in the testes and, in small amounts, from the adrenal cortex. Responsible for much of the sex drive in both males and females.

Anemia.   Low levels of hemoglobin (iron) in the blood and/or an insufficient red blood cell count. Reduces the amount of oxygen that the blood can carry to the working muscles.

Angina (angina pectoris).   Chest pain, occurring during exercise, that is often associated with a narrowing of the arteries and consequent restriction blood flow to the heart muscle itself.

Anorexia.   A loss of appetite often experienced by females trying to lose weight. If extended over a longer period of time, a condition called anorexia nervosa can lead to extreme weight loss.

Basal metabolic rate (BMR).   The lowest level of energy expenditure when the body is at complete rest. At that time we are using about 3.5 $ml0_2/kg/min$ and burning around 0.5 to 0.7 calories per minute.

Blood glucose.   The amount of sugar in the blood. Normal range from 80 to 100 mg percent. Lower than 60 to 70 may result in hypoglycemia; scores over 120 to 140 may be considered hyperglycemia and often is an indication of early diabetes.

Blood pressure.   Blood pressure is represented by two numbers— for example, 120/70. The top number is called systolic blood pressure and is the maximum pressure that is exerted on the arteries as the heart beats and pushes out blood. The lower, smaller number is the diastolic blood pressure and is the amount of pressure that remains in the arteries between heartbeats.

Bradycardia.   An unusually slow heart rate, probably below 60 beats per minute. It is usually considered very healthy, and can be lowered by following long-term exercise programs.

Calorie.   A measure of work and energy. For example, at rest you burn off less than 1 calorie per minute. Walking around a room burns off 1 to 2 calories per minute. Vigorous exercise uses 4 to 10 calories per minute, and very vigorous exercise will burn off approximately 15 calories per minute (3,500 calories represents 1 pound of body fat).

Carbohydrate. A chemical compound containing carbon, hydrogen and oxygen. Carbohydrates are basic foodstuffs found in starches, cellulose and sugars.

Cardiac. Referring to the heart.

Cardiac output. The amount of blood pumped out of the heart each minute. The cardiac output is the product of the number of beats per minute times the stroke volume (amount of blood pumped out of the heart during each beat, usually around 70 ml or 2.5 oz of blood).

Carotid sinus. A portion of the carotid artery that divides into two separate branches. Touching or pressing this artery may change the heart rate and is not recommended for heart rate monitoring.

Catecholamines. Chemical compound secreted by the adrenal medulla. These chemical hormones include epinephrine and norepinephrine (adrenaline and noradrenaline are the man-made chemical correspondents).

Cholesterol. A fatty substance combined with protein to form a molecule called a lipoprotein. For example, the low-density lipoprotein (LDL) molecule contains about 50 percent cholesterol. Cholesterol is essential for life and is found in the various tissues, including the sex organs. It is produced in the liver as well as in other cells of the body. Elevated levels have been associated with increased risk of coronary heart disease.

Chronic. Referring to something that occurs for a long period of time. For example, a disease lasting for six months may be considered chronic.

Conditioning. A change in physical fitness resulting from participation in exercise programs.

Continuous work. Exercise performed from start to finish without rest periods. Fifteen minutes of exercise with one or two quick stops for a six-second pulse count would be considered continuous work.

Coordination. Movement in a smooth, organized manner.

Coronary arteries. Blood vessels that exit from the aorta and branch out to supply blood and oxygen back to the heart muscle.

Dehydration. Loss of essential body fluids through sweating or lack of fluid intake.

Diaphragm. A major muscle responsible for breathing.

Diastolic (blood pressure). See Blood pressure.

Diuretic. A substance that increases the frequency of urination, thus providing a loss of body fluids.

Dyspnea. Labored or forced breathing.

ECG. A graphic record of the electrical activities of the heart (sometimes EKG).

Edema. Overloading with fluid.

Electrolytes. Electrically charged atoms found in the blood. Examples are sodium and potassium, which are essential for proper metabolism.

Endurance. Ability to withstand fatigue. Includes cardiovascular and muscular endurance.

Ergometer. A device that can measure work, such as a bicycle or treadmill.

Evaporation. Changing a liquid into a vapor.

Exercise. Any form of physical activity.

Exercise prescription. An individual exercise program which outlines the frequency, intensity, duration and type of exercise.

Fat. A digestible food composed of glycerol and fatty acids. Stored in the fat cells of the body. When excess fat, carbohydrates or protein is ingested, it is transformed into fat and stored in fat cells throughout the body.

Fatigue. Inability to maintain a certain level of physical performance due to a lack of fitness or exercising at a very high intensity.

Glucose. Blood sugar transported in the blood is utilized when you exercise vigorously. A major source of nutrients for the brain.

Glycogen. A form of glucose that is stored for emergency use in the liver and muscles.

Growth hormone. A hormone manufactured in the pituitary gland and associated with growth, among other things. Growth hormone increases the amount of fatty acids and glucose in the blood. Growth hormone levels increase with exercise.

Heart rate. The number of times the heart beats each minute.

Heat stress. Performing activities in excessive environmental heat.

Humidity. Measurement of the amount of moisture in the air.

Hypercholesterolemia. Elevated amounts of cholesterol in the blood. (See also Cholesterol.) Optimal levels less than 200 mg percent.

Hypertension. Often referred to as high blood pressure; usually scores of 140/90 mmHg or above. It may eventually lead to heart, kidney and brain damage.

Hyperthermia. Overheating of the body caused by a lack of fluid or exercising in high temperatures or while wearing rubberized suits.

Hypertrophy. An increase in the size of the muscles usually due to increasing work or exercise.

Hyperventilation. Rapid and deep breathing which frequently occurs as a result of exercise. Also, increased breathing rate above levels necessary for normal function. May cause dizziness, fainting, and decrease normal carbon dioxide levels in the blood.

Hypoglycemia. Low blood sugar; less than 70 to 80 mg percent.

Hypotension. Low blood pressure. Less than 90/60 mmHg.

Hypoxia. Insufficient oxygen in the blood or body tissue. One sign of hypoxia is bluish skin or lips.

Intermittent work. Exercise performed with alternate periods of rest. The opposite is continuous work.

Interval training. A type of intermittent work used by runners and other athletes to improve "wind." Consists of alternating sessions of fast runs and recovery sessions for specific intervals.

Ischemia. A lack of adequate blood to a muscle or tissue. Ischemia often refers to an obstruction of the blood vessel supplying blood to the heart.

Isometric contraction. A static muscle contraction in which the limb does not move. An example would be pushing against an immovable wall as hard as you can.

Isotonic contraction. A moving contraction. An example would be lifting a five-pound weight from the table.

Jumping. Various physical activities performed on rebounding equipment. The activities include bouncing, jumping, turning, twisting and kicking, all done in a rhythmic manner.

Kilogram (kg).   A metric unit of weight equal to 2.2 pounds.

Lactic acid.   A waste product resulting from vigorous anaerobic exercise.

Ligaments.   A tough connective band of tissue that binds bones together at the joints to maintain stability.

Lipid.   Fat or fatlike substance.

Lipoprotein.   A molecule containing fat and protein.

Liter.   A metric unit of capacity nearly equal to 1 quart.

Maximal oxygen consumption (VO_2 max).   The absolute maximum rate at which oxygen can be consumed during one minute of maximum exercise. It is the best index of total body fitness and endurance. It is often called aerobic fitness, aerobic power, maximal oxygen uptake or maximal oxygen consumption.

Mental practice.   Imagining or mentally rehearsing an activity or event.

Met.   The equivalent of approximately 1.2 calories per minute, which is measured during rest in a sitting position. The oxygen equivalent of one met is 3.5 $ml0_2$/kg/min. If you determine that your fitness level is 35 $ml0_2$/kg/min, your maximum working level would be the equivalent of 10 mets.

Metabolism.   All of the chemical changes resulting in caloric burn-off within the body.

Milliliter (ml).   One-thousandth of a liter. (See also Liter.)

Minerals.   Inorganic compounds necessary for proper body function, including calcium, iron, iodine, potassium, sodium and phosphorus.

Mitochondria.   Subcellular bodies located in the muscle and other cells and in which most of the body's energy is manufactured from sugar, fats and oxygen.

Mixed diet.   Normal diet containing appropriate amounts of unprocessed carbohydrates, nonsaturated fat and low-fat protein.

Norepinephrine.   A chemical secreted by the sympathetic nerve endings and by the adrenal medulla that increases heart rate and blood pressure.

Nutrition. The body's ability to take in, digest and assimilate foods.

Obesity. An excess amount of body fat, usually representing 20 percent above standard norm. Above 30 percent for women and 22 percent for men.

Overfat. The state of having excessive body fat; usually characterized by having fat scores above 24 percent for women and above 17 percent for men.

Overload. Placing stress on the muscles above what is normally experienced.

Oxygen debt. The amount of oxygen used during an exercise bout above the normal resting consumption. After exercise, you continue to breathe more rapidly in order to reoxygenate your system, "paying back" the oxygen debt.

Plasma. The fluid portion of the blood, not including the red blood cells.

Protein. Organic compound of amino acids. Forms the muscle tissue and is found in animal and vegetable matter.

Pulse. The pressure of blood expanding the arteries during each heartbeat. Counting the pulse is the same as counting the heart rate.

Pulse pressure. The mathematical difference between the systolic and diastolic blood pressures (130/80 mmHg = pulse pressure of 50 mmHg).

Respiration. During breathing, the exchange of gases within the lung and tissue. The number of breaths per minute averages around 12. During moderate exercise, the rate is about 20, and at maximal exercise, the rate may reach 30 breaths per minute.

Saturated fat. Fat chemically constructed so that it cannot absorb any more hydrogen. These fats are solid at room temperature and are of animal origin, such as meat, milk, butter, cheese, etc.

Sclerosis. Hardening of material usually due to the accumulation of cholesterol and fiber tissues in the arteries.

Second wind. A physiological feeling that comes during rather vigorous exercise and is characterized by a sudden lessening of the feeling of distress or fatigue.

Skin fold. The measure of the thickness of the skin and underlying fat.

Steady state. A state of exercise in which the amount of oxygen taken in is matched with the amount of oxygen needed for the working muscles. This can also be termed aerobic state.

Stitch in the side.   A sharp pain at the side or under the rib cage resulting from vigorous unaccustomed exercise.

Strength.   The ability of the muscle to exert maximal force.

Stroke volume.   The amount of blood pumped each heartbeat (at rest, stroke volume is about 70 ml of blood).

Submaximal exercise.   Exercise at less than maximal intensity or duration.

Testosterone.   The dominant male androgen. A hormone, secreted by the testes in the male, that is responsible for the male's sex drive. Testosterone levels are reduced by aging and can be improved by restricting alcohol consumption, eliminating the smoking of tobacco and marijuana, and increasing exercise.

Tonus.   Muscle firmness in the absence of voluntary contraction.

Training.   A program of exercise which will result in improved skills, strength and endurance.

Triglycerides.   A fat consisting of three fatty acids and glycerol. It is a normal circulating fat that has a secondary effect in the development of heart disease.

Vein.   A vessel that transports blood toward the heart.

Ventilation.   The movement of air in and out of the lungs. (*See also* Respiration.)

Vitamins.   Organic nutrients necessary for normal metabolic reactions to occur. Vitamins are classified as "water soluble" or "fat soluble."

Weight control.   Maintaining proper weight with adequate exercise and nutritional balance.

Weight training.   Progressive-resistance exercises using various weights for resistance.

Work.   The product of force times distance.